GOD

FROM CONCEPT TO LIFESTYLE

FIRST

MARCOS A DE CAMARGO E SILVA

GOD FIRST, from Concept to Lifestyle!

Also in Portuguese: "DEUS PRIMEIRO, do Conceito ao Estilo de Vida!"

Original Text: @marcosacamargo, 2024

You are now part of a very large family. Even though we talk about thousands of people on this earth, I like to think that each reader is part of my experiences. That's why I want to treat you with love and respect, always giving you, my best. This is my commitment to God and to you.

INTRODUCTION 7

1 - GOD FIRST, FROM CONCEPT TO LIFESTYLE! 13

2 - ONE MORE DEGREE 43

3 – YOUR VALUES, MY VALUES 56

4 - FROM ACHAN TO GEHAZI IN EACH ONE OF US! HOW TO GET OUT OF THIS. 75

5 - PARADIGMS AND OTHER TRUTHS 88

6 – WHOSE IDEA WAS IT? 104

7 - TITHING, MUCH MORE THAN A BOGEYMAN! 114

8 - TRUE PROSPERITY 174

9 - I'VE LEARNED THE CONCEPT, I WANT TO LIVE THE REALITY! 213

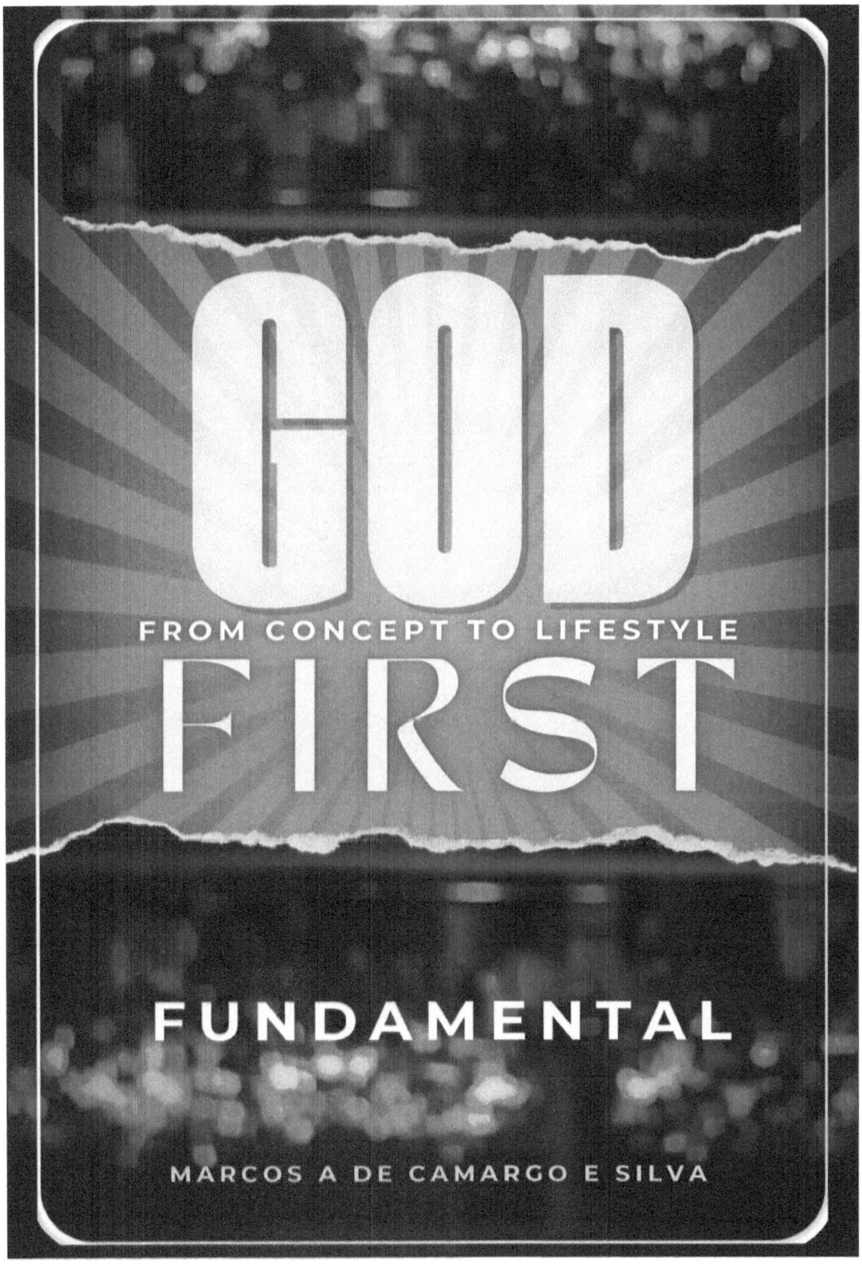

GOD
FROM CONCEPT TO LIFESTYLE
FIRST
FUNDAMENTAL
MARCOS A DE CAMARGO E SILVA

Fundamental

As I write this introduction, while Israel seeks to find the hostages taken since October 7, 2023, we see the nations that support it and those that revolt against it. We also observe Iran's first direct attack on Israel. During the launch of some 300 drones and more than a hundred missiles, all were fully identified in the air and destroyed, thanks to war technology. In these months of relentless killing and fighting, we reflect on God's command to pray for the peace of Jerusalem.

...

We thus understood that our obedience cannot depend on the obedience of others. My understanding of the Word and my attitude towards it must not be tied to circumstances. Whether we understand it or not, I'm talking about principles. Our obedience to God's Word cannot depend on current circumstances and our mentality must pursue the timeless and infinite, because it is focused on the Eternal.

"Do not conform to the pattern of this world but be transformed by the renewing of your mind. Then you will be able to test

There are moments in life that stay with you forever. I have had, and still have, wonderful experiences with my children that occasionally make me smile as I remember what we experienced and how much we gained from it. I remember when I had come home from school and was sitting in the living room in Tulsa, Oklahoma, and suddenly my two daughters came in crying because their little fingers were hurting so much. I took off their gloves, coats and hats, cleaned off the snow that was still on them, and warmed them up with a hug and a hot chocolate. The little boots damp with snow and sand that would soon be worn again were put aside while they warmed up, now calmer and happier again. Whenever it snowed, we chose a place to slide down the mountain and these are moments we never forget.

I remember taking my daughters for a walk along the waterfront in Bridgeport, Connecticut, where we moved. We'd watch the big ships passing along the coast in the direction of New York. Among so many memories, one stand out because it is relevant to what I invite you to explore in this reading.

I taught my three girls and my son to ride bicycles, using a gentle and fun method that prepared them for the freedom that comes with mastering the art of pedaling. The family would get together and we'd go to a park, where the wide lawn provided space and some trees served as obstacles, teaching them how to swerve and stay focused.

The process began with me pushing the bike and asking each of them to step on the pedal with force. Each child reacted differently to the challenge, but they were all motivated by the reward that was soon to come. After a few minutes, the skill of pedaling was conquered. Enjoying the rhythm, I gradually decreased the force of the push. Soon, balance became evident, and I instructed them to look ahead, to the horizon, focusing on the goal. Then I'd say: "Now, get on the bike again and 'draw' an 8 on the ground!" The rest was pure fun, full of laughter, band-aids and bandages.

That's how your journey through this book might be. One day at a time. We will go step by step, bringing understanding of the whole context and, in the end, when you have mastered the art of believing in God above all else, you will not only fulfill what is necessary, but you will enjoy the abundant life that is promised and prepared for us by the Creator. God has established small methods so that, if we are courageous and willing, we will certainly achieve the long-awaited success.

Use this time as an investment! Feel free to investigate the facts presented here. Not everything will be delved into exhaustively, as I hope to bring the essence of the points necessary for individual knowledge and improvement, believing that the Holy Spirit completes all reasoning and logic in favor of the Kingdom of God. There is nothing better than living in love with the truth, because peace of heart comes when we believe and live the Word more than our own human wills and desires.

We will discover how God's purpose makes us happy, reconciled, triumphant and prosperous people. So don't accept being just another skeptic, atheist or critic, and rush to delve - in your own time - into the fundamentals of reason; invest time in what adds up and brings results.

Biblical criticism and discussion is important and necessary when it is done from a heart and intelligence that is focused on a real quest that makes sense to pursue. This, in fact, is called wisdom. We'll walk through the concepts, but my focus is to help you arrive at the lifestyle with God always first. That's why I want to ask you:

- Has the path you've chosen worked out or does it just seem right?
- Does the search, the family tradition, the faith you follow bring permanent results or do you live on a rollercoaster of demands just trying to make everyone happy?
- With security or insecurity, how do people perceive you?

It would be good to stop and investigate what is going on there, in the depths of your feelings. If you haven't figured out how to do it yet, ask God, think and present your question and the answer will come. I can guarantee that something good will be presented; your mind and heart will receive something, and you will be able to think, reflect, change, be transformed by the power that dwells in the Word! This is my goal, my target!

These reflections, added to your own considerations, will provide enough opportunity to transform you from who you are today to someone much better, more complete and healthier, in all areas of your life.

On this journey of reading, we will certainly clarify points that you have never thought about and may not even agree with. I don't expect to stick to my opinions or my guesses, the results of which can be embarrassing. Human justice has already been proven to fail, and the Bible itself states that the aroma is not good, it smells like filthy rags. Better than my opinions is to bring and make diagnoses. Just as we look to doctors for an answer to a possible pain and a possible treatment, the Word of God must be sought in order to treat our heart with excellence - our inner self - everything that God sees; through the Word the answer is revealed to us, which comes as an accurate diagnosis enhanced by the power of the Holy Spirit in us.

"My people are destroyed from lack of knowledge". [Hosea 4.6]

The invitation is made... so is the challenge! I don't expect to put you at ease, as if it were just another weekend read.

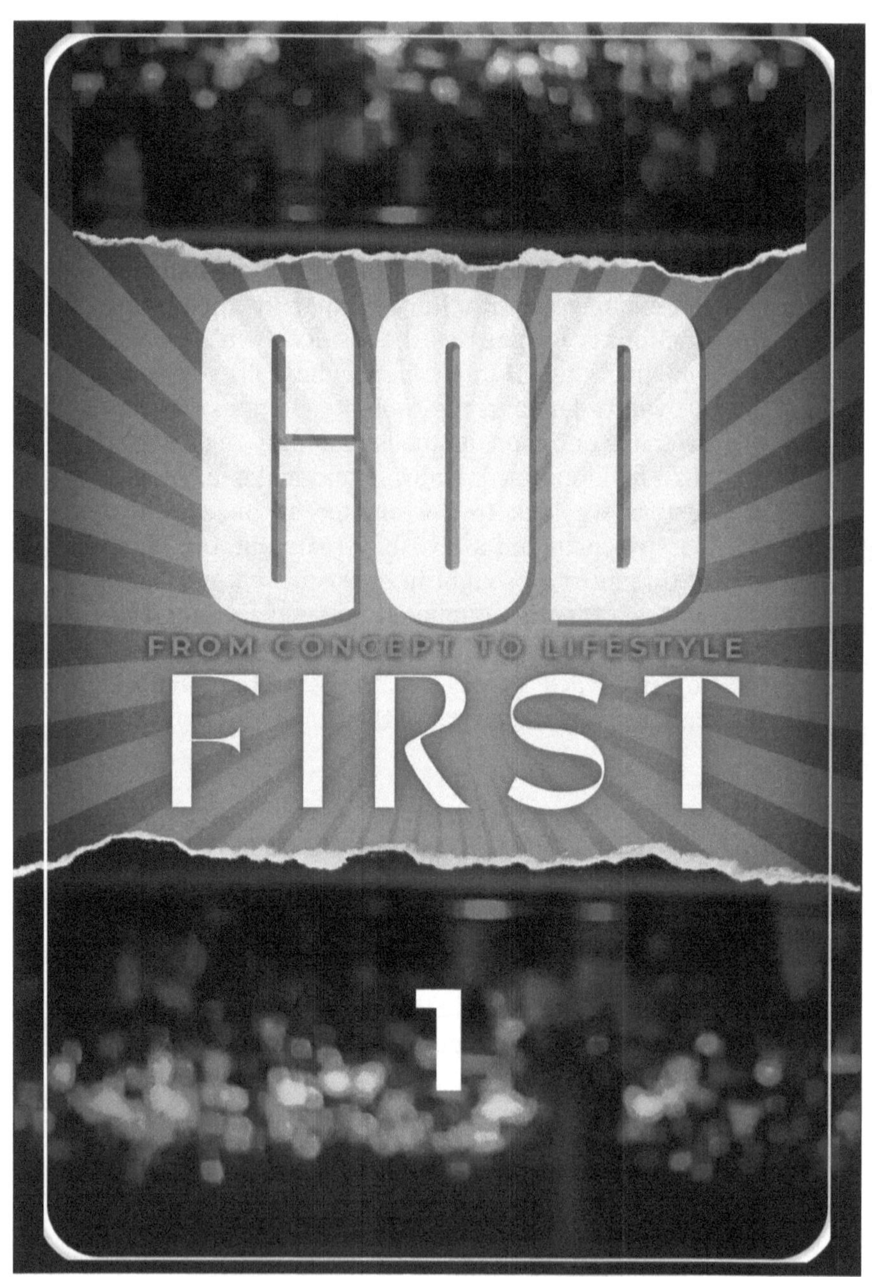

GOD
FIRST
FROM CONCEPT TO LIFESTYLE
1

1 - GOD FIRST, FROM CONCEPT TO LIFESTYLE!

""This is what the Lord says— Israel's King and Redeemer, the Lord Almighty: I am the first and I am the last; apart from me there is no God.". [Isaiah 44.6]

"But seek first his kingdom and his righteousness, and all these things will be given to you as well.". [Matthew 6.33]

We are constantly ministered to by the Word to remind us of what it means to understand and heed a principle, as opposed to being in a place where our understanding rules us. To explain: as we read the Word from the Old Testament to the end of the New Testament, God repeatedly teaches us about principles related to our lives and finances, and this certainly includes nations, organizations and people. The principles and statutes that serve as the foundation for peace and prosperity in every sense have been sidelined by the culture and society in which we live.

When we read biblical passages, we discover that God seeks our hearts; it's not about money and it's not about power. We constantly hear about generosity, and one of the references we see is the

Macedonians who, even without conditions, gave everything they had to help advance the Kingdom, the early church and the gospel in general.

Even earlier, in Old Testament times, David wanted to build the temple, but God said: *"You can't build the temple because your hands are dirty with blood."* However, David had such a passion for this work for God that he decided to set aside his possessions so that his son could build the temple. He extended an invitation to the faithful to voluntarily bring their possessions and wealth for the future construction of the temple. David was deeply touched by the people's response and said a beautiful prayer of thanks to God for the lives of those people who understood the purpose of his heart.

God wants us to give with joy and a willing heart, not out of embarrassment. In Malachi, we find a matter of principle: if you trust in God and hand over what is yours to Him, rest assured that He will take care of you and provide for your needs. The Bible talks about many principles related to finances, almost like a tool for us to train and test our intent in God. It's as if finances were gym equipment. To get strong, there's no point in sitting on the sofa; you must use weights and do exercises.

Finances work for us as a piece of equipment, a tool for exercising a generous, willing heart that trusts in God and understands what the Kingdom is. This Kingdom of God is still in full swing among the nations and in the hearts of every person on earth, a tool for exercising our obedience and faith. I mentioned the issue of war at the beginning of this book. We saw that Iran had announced yet another attack on Israel and we immediately began to pray for the peace of Jerusalem. The great truth is that, from a geopolitical point of view, we understand little and have little information. Even if we search, we won't have all the answers, but everything is connected to God's plans for humanity. The health and prosperity of nations has to do with God's heart for all of humanity.

We won't discuss here what the level of reason is between the sides, and it doesn't matter because there is one word that doesn't change and it's in the Bible and, regardless of whether we understand it or not, we know that God has given us a commandment: "Pray for the peace of Jerusalem." What I do know is that I need to exercise my faith and obedience, doing what the Bible tells me to do, doing my part!

Our daily religiousness!

The news we read, the thoughts we have or hear on the radio, newspapers and in the media in general, often consume us to the point where we almost lose focus and hope that something good might happen in our lives. So, let's find out what people in general have to say about some important points of Christianity.

Is your reading time an investment? Then choose to be curious and optimistic, knowing that there are good and bad professionals everywhere, good and bad teachers, good and bad believers, and yes, leaders who don't deserve the honor of occupying their positions.

I have learned that I should never dismiss ideas or people, whether they are simple or complex, young or old. I prefer to reflect with empathy and assess whether I can walk through and discuss the ideas put on the table; often questioning, confronting, opening myself up, but always giving my all. Even so, at times I give myself the chance to keep my distance. And if you, the reader, don't want to be confronted or aren't willing to put your paradigms on the line, ask yourself if you should go ahead. I hope you do.

My choices, my options, my will!

You might say: "What nonsense! How can anyone feel at ease if they're not encouraged to read these chapters?"

The fact is that not everyone is ready to change their life. Perhaps financial comfort has already been achieved and satisfaction has been reached. Perhaps relationships are going very well, and this tends to generate a comfort zone. There are also those who are more reserved in their world of absolute truths and don't allow room for reason, especially when it comes to the excellent principles that flow from Scripture. But we will discuss many of these points here.

Our discussion will be around the divine principles related to God being first in life, in business or in whatever leadership one is part of. This requires more strategic thinking in terms of where to put your efforts. Biblical principles are blessing and encourage us to deliver more than we gather for ourselves. You will understand principles that will broaden your view of finances, time, mission and much more. It's impossible to think that, in the times we live in, anyone would just want to accumulate, as if that were the most important thing in life. But what impact will this have? And how will our living affect the people we live with?

Just another movie?

In 2024 we experienced the Paris Olympics, an event marked by great records and victories by athletes, but which will also be remembered for the depressing images of its opening ceremony, which featured ludicrous scenes with obvious anti-Christian overtones. It is events like these that challenge us to reflect on the values we promote and the messages we convey. While we celebrate the achievements of athletes, it is also essential to consider the cultural and spiritual context in which these events take place.

Exactly one hundred years earlier, another Olympics took place in Paris, recalled in the movie Chariots of Fire. Released in 1981 and directed by

Hugh Hudson, the film is an inspiring drama, accompanied by the iconic soundtrack composed by the Greek Vangelis, which has become the official anthem of many marathons and athletes around the world. Competitions in schools and clubs are still rocked by this unforgettable piece.

The film, which is still worth watching today, shows the preparation of the Great Britain Olympic athletics team for the 1924 Olympic Games in Paris. Two characters appear as athletes: Eric Liddell (Ian Charleson), a Scottish missionary who ran out of devotion to God, and Harold Abrahams (Ben Cross), a Jew who had recently become rich and wanted to prove his ability to Cambridge society.

What is striking is Liddell's devotion, an athlete who ran using only his natural talent, with energy and showcasing the beauty of the mountains where he trained. Both went through the qualifiers without any problems, until one of Liddell's qualifiers was scheduled for Sunday. He refused to compete because it was a day he set aside to worship God. Noticing the situation, a nobleman offered Liddell his place in the 400-meter race, which would take place on Saturday. Of course, this attracted attention. How could someone waste such an opportunity because of their faith? Something that for many people wouldn't make a difference, for him it did, because it was the foundation for everything he believed in.

You could interpret this as mere religiosity, since he could go to the race, win and come back the following Sunday to be in church, just the same. Nothing would change. However, what we see here is just a portrait of the decisions that take place beforehand, in each person's heart. His Jewish friend, Abrahams, also won his race the next day. However, it was Liddell's example that was marked by the choice he made, showing determination and courage not to give in to something he believed was wrong. He wanted to serve God first.

Choices and legacies

People make choices all the time. My brother, Dr. Osmar Camargo, and his wife Olinda, both PhDs in Marriage Counseling, have dedicated their lives to the mission field in the United States, Japan and are currently counselors in Portugal. Osmar, in addition to his dedication to missionary ministry, was a top athlete in his youth. He and I trained karate at a gym at Sacred Heart University in Bridgeport, Connecticut.

The athlete and the teacher

He was my teacher and a highly recognized athlete among competitors. Whenever he had the chance, Osmar competed in challenging championships in the United States. He was respected by everyone as an athlete, winning many competitions in Connecticut, New York and New Jersey. His attacks and defenses were a reference point for the more than three hundred students at the academies who practiced the technique we used. His fights were watched with great anticipation, providing technical learning for everyone.

Commitment to the faith

At the Saturday and Sunday competitions, he was there whenever he could. But something about his behavior always caught the eye. If the competition took place on a Sunday, he would warn the team: *"I have an appointment in the afternoon at my church. Will this competition be long?"*. His friends couldn't understand how such a skilled wrestler, with all the conditions for victory and medals, would consider giving up his fighting just to go to church. Once, almost at the end of a competition, he put aside the trophy to honor what resonated most strongly in his life, returned to his town and took part in his commitment to God.

A powerful testimony

It may seem silly, an act of pure religiosity, but I was there on one of the occasions when his faith was tested. We were together at what was to be the last annual meeting with the academies of the states, where hundreds of athletes were taking part. Unexpectedly, he asked his master to excuse him, took the floor and spoke loud and clear to everyone present: *"I want to say a big thank you to my karate masters who, for all these years, have taught me this art that has inspired me and made me grow as a person. However, as of today, by my choice, I'm leaving this art that I love so much to dedicate myself to something even greater; here are these weapons, my spear, my rapier, my sash, my uniform, my technique. I'm going to fight for something I love even more: Jesus! I'm going to be ordained as a pastor and I want to dedicate myself entirely, spirit, soul and body, and I invite each of you to get to know Jesus, as I know Him!"*

Audience reaction

Moved, upset, surprised and proud, all kinds of feelings and impressions were expressed that day. That scene will remain etched in the memory of hundreds of people, a powerful testimony of someone who serves God without reservation. We didn't have television or as many photos as at the French Olympics, but it was another day when someone had the courage to put God first in their life.

Liddell's example and Osmar Camargo's story reminds us that the choices we make shape not only our lives, but also the legacy we leave for generations to come. But it takes courage to make choices that honor God and inspire others to follow the same path. By prioritizing our faith and our commitment to the Lord, we will build a legacy that transcends time and impacts lives.

Lifestyle is not fashion

Humanity's greatest difficulties have been its failure to comply with the laws established by the Creator from the beginning. We were not thrown onto the earth without any plan, direction or purpose; God breathes life into every mother's womb, and the intention has always been multiplication and abundance. We will discuss some of these bases and concepts from different perspectives, which add up to God's wishes for humanity. If we want to live well and better, if we hope to have a fulfilling life, the advice is to respect what was already established before we got here.

For example, the law of free will, which most of the time, perhaps out of ignorance, has been confused with other behaviors that cognitive science seeks to impose on people, without for some reason being able to prove its non-existence and action in absolutely every human being. "In the majority of societies and cultures spread across the earth, free will has been considered a characteristic or capacity innate to human beings, with a unique and special value." We have fallen victim to thinking that is quite contrary to what we believe and what is presented to us as a legacy and responsibility in the Word of God.

The concept and principle of free will is closely linked to other laws, such as that of giving and receiving. The next step, based on this understanding, is what we do with the constant information we receive: do we want to obey and live the Word as a lifestyle, or do we mold ourselves to what fashion dictates? For me, this is exactly the question where many stop - perhaps the majority - because they are only consumed by what has been studied but fail to learn how to exercise these concepts, transforming them into a lifestyle.

Small gestures, small behaviors, attitudes and desires are expressions of our understanding and practice of such blessing principles that are exercised daily. Many of the biblical aspects we deal with confront and contradict everything that modern society offers. Giving? The Bible has already established the principle: *"It is more blessed to give than to receive!"* That's the word that comes from the mouth of God!

I remember the school I attended as a child in Brasília, Brazil, a public school that still brings back fond memories. It was common to see joy and noise in the classroom; we were all happy and noisy children. Children are naturally talkative and don't pay much attention to what's important, because they talk, talk and talk. One day, while the boys and girls were playing and talking so loudly and uncontrollably - and I was certainly one of those who contributed to the racket. The disrespect was clear and there wasn't much to be done, as there is today in every classroom; after all, for children, this question of principles has never been so natural, until the teacher, in a moment of agony and desperation, shouted: *"Stop, listen to me! I want to talk!"*. Then, frightened by the volume of our teacher's voice, we all stopped, and respect suddenly existed again and lasted from that moment of "imminent danger". Her word was worth it!

Later, my parents enrolled me in another school where; to speak, we had to wait, raise our hands and wait for permission, otherwise we would be grounded for good. In short, I learned to appreciate when someone has something to say, and I realized that both speaking and listening must be observed, because there are principles that, if not correctly observed, will only be recorded conceptually.

Some years later, when I was young and newly married and studying abroad, I met Tim Stemple and Bernardo Snelgrove, a friend who had lived in Brazil for many years. I met him again at the home of Evangelist Dave Roberson. That evening, Bernardo, much more experienced and clearly seeking to pass on principles that I could invest in, called me into the corner of the room and said: *"Marcos, you are starting out in life, and you have the privilege of being amid very important people, who certainly speak the Word of God with authority. So, keep it in your heart and write down everything you hear. One day you will understand the value of this habit"*. His words have stayed with me to this day, even after more than 40 years. Today I am very grateful to have accepted the challenge to value what people say, as well as being able to go back in time in my notes and remember much of what I learned from listening and observing.

At the end of the 1990s, I had the privilege of translating Dave Roberson himself here in Brazil, among many others who became friends, such as Evangelist T.L. Osborn, when we worked together for a week conference in São Paulo. A small man in stature, soft-spoken, but with unparalleled authority. Not only did the word he ministered in those days speak to me, but also the small notebook he held with great care. There were little snippets of his words, verses that he pasted between his thoughts on the pages he looked at as he spoke. Before he began his last day, in the Portuguesa sports hall, he and I sat in a corner of the room that overlooked the main stage and I listened to him attentively, then I asked him to pray for me and my home. I received a word from God for my family which was deeply marked inside me.

The word and authority that comes from heaven

If we stop to give some value to people who touch us with beautiful and often wise words, even if they are just to get our attention, how much greater the privilege of knowing that we can listen to God's voice, hear His voice and come to live what is whispered in our spirit - imagine the joy of the authors who were inspired to compose the books of the Bible, without perhaps ever realizing that they left us a wonderful legacy just because they obeyed. Think of the grandeur of the universe that has surrounded us since creation. God opening his voice and declaring to the whole universe, from chapter 1 in Genesis to the close in chapter 22 of Revelation. *"In the beginning God created the heavens and the earth"* and all he had to do was open his mouth and speak. The galaxy stopped and made itself available, the angels were attentive and ready to act, nature trembled, the abyss, the waters, and even the 'nothingness' that was about to exist, everything and everyone turned to respond to what the I Am had to speak and decree.

And so, God spoke! And that was good! The Prophet Jeremiah, for example, chosen by God to warn the kingdom of Judah of its imminent destruction, did not begin his journey until he had received an express command from God. Look what he said: *"The word of the Lord has come to me!"*. He discovered how much God knew him from the womb and even before he was born. It took a word from God for everything in his life to start happening.

Another person we see listening and exposing what God has said is the psalmist David, who tells his story in which his heart reveals the commitment and direction of his life and that of all of us. He says: *"O Lord, you search my heart and know everything about me"*. It's another song by the psalmist that demonstrates the transparency of every aspect of his being, his habits and behavior, and his character so that they can be examined by God. Here we also see declared both the omniscience and omnipotence of the Lord, who comes, through His Word, to give us the comfort we so much expect from Him.

The 'God First' concept

There is a well-defined concept of the Word, characterized by the breath - Hebrew: ruach - of the Lord. Every time God speaks, we can look to see three clear manifestations:

1.   **Generation and Creation**: He generates what needs to be created, using as raw material what He Himself has created or what can come from nothing. The earth, therefore, was formless and empty. He created and established the balance of earth, sky and sea, of animals, vegetation, fish; everything came in the order given by the mouth of God.

2.   **Giving of Life**: He gives life. While humanity invests and spends billions and billions of dollars and euros to survive and try to stay healthy, even if only for a short time, God uses just one breath, and something comes into existence. He created man, gave him life, and from him, created woman. Everything God made was original. He didn't use recycled material or raw materials from elsewhere. He only needed to declare and, out of *nothing* - literally, from Hebrew: *bara* - everything we see was created.

3.   **Transformation**: He transforms things and hearts. Here again, God's manifestation is evident in the miracles and wonders we read about, witness and experience. In the New Testament, in Luke 2, the Angel presented himself to Mary and delivered the Word that God had

declared. The angel of the Lord was the bearer of a Word that came to create, to generate life and to transform all of humanity's perceptions of the supernatural up to that point. The word came from God in the voice of an angel, with the Creator's peculiar creativity. This immediately generated life in Mary's womb, and her interior began a unique transformation so that the very Son of God, Jesus, would come from her.

So, it is with people's lives; they will speak and hear thousands of words every day. Words that reach their ears and present themselves from various sources such as the internet, newspapers, apps, laughter, advice and conversations. Everyone can receive them via spirit, soul or body. Once again, culture is in transition and in constant search of new concepts and ideas that feed the whole being. What we hear most these days is the search for Artificial Intelligence (AI) and, from there, we will be able to listen and learn anything. And the question that makes us stop and reflect is how much of this is supernatural and transformational?

From all these sources of information, however, we know that only the word inspired by the breath of the Spirit comes with the supernatural power to create, bring life and transform. And the result of this is that the person believes and receives it, being a divine and supernatural inspiration, but only because it came directly from God. It is the experience of having a word that has been blown into your interior and you simply interpret it, obviously in line with the Scriptures, which is the voice of God, transmitted and influencing, that impacts us.

Perspective on the Pandemic

Francis Chan, a renowned pastor from California, after years of dedication and planting one of the most respected churches in the United States, suddenly, upon hearing the voice of God, left his comfort and, with his family, went to Hong Kong and other places outside the U.S.A., obeying an order from heaven that reflected his discomfort with the things he was doing, even though they were seen as a success. A few years of experience passed, and he and his family eventually returned, now with a new focus and outlook on all that God had spoken to them.

During the pandemic, he brought a quick online message to believers and non-believers alike, entitled *"Perspective in the Pandemic: The Leader's Check"*, where Pastor Chan warned those watching him to repent and consider the possibility that, when the pandemic is over, we shouldn't go back to the pattern of "church as usual". *"What if God is taking us to a different place?"* was Francis Chan's question. *"Many of us are anxious to get back to normal soon. I hope your anxiety isn't just because you want to get back to your many activities,"* he concluded.

Human nature tends to return to its place of comfort whenever it has the chance to do so. The pandemic has given man the opportunity to look again at the center and reason of his purpose with God, offering yet another chance for humanity to rekindle the understanding that God must be first in all life situations. A few years on from the pandemic, it seems that humanity, unfortunately, hasn't learned much from it. So, what value do we place on the faith we claim to live and what do we do with it? Failing to respond to what is greatest and truest is the same as forgetting who should and always will be first in our lives. The most important thing here is the responsibility we are given and the response we give when we hear God speaking.

End times?

In this way, par excellence, Chan emphatically called out to his friends that this moment was fundamentally relevant for them to re-evaluate their lives and realize the level of their relationship with God. When a virus threatens to take you and those you love, it brings up the perspective of Scripture, which says:

> *"Take heed now, you who say, 'Today or tomorrow we will go to such and such a city, and spend a year there, and trade, and make a profit. You do not know what will happen tomorrow. What is your life? You are only like mist that appears for a moment and then vanishes."* [4]

Chan also shared about a friend who decided to leave his wife for another woman during the time of the global pandemic. His reaction was one of disbelief: *"Do you have the courage to do that now?"*. How difficult it is to understand that people can choose to continue in sin even during a time of such uncertainty as the one we are living in. How often, during the circumstances that beset us and prevent us from thinking properly, we are led to forget everything that has already been spoken and sown to us every time we read and meditate on the Scriptures.

It's possible that not only the pandemic, but our experiences and what we see in this society are the beginning of the end, in the face of the fulfillment of millennial prophecies! There is agreement when we say that God is doing something new like we have never had the chance to experience in our entire lives... and this makes us feel that we are entering a new season. It makes us stop and re-evaluate our behavior and delivery as Christians! Am I listening to God's voice? Is he first in my life right now? What do I hope to see happen through me; will I be part of this divine purpose?

Within this understanding, if we really are in the end times, the last thing we need to focus on is the accumulation of goods, which brings us back to Luke 12, where the rich man prioritizes storing goods and food in his barns. How many times have we consciously caught ourselves storing and piling up possessions, which we eventually discover are stored somewhere without any need for use. Our lives, like the rich man's, can be taken unexpectedly. We learn from this parable that we can have riches, and there's nothing to stop us getting there. But it's also a matter of life and death.

By being generous with what we have received from God, we will achieve life; otherwise, death. This is no time to hoard!

The voice of the obedient prophet

Another voice that impacted Brazil was that of Dr. Don Lynch - my dear teacher and eternal friend, who left us memories of a man fully confident in God's provision and grace. For more than 16 years, I was continually amazed by his sensitivity in digging into the Word and bringing out what many had not yet had the opportunity to see. He had this absurd clarity of receiving and perceiving God's voice. Every word was always announced with the peculiar authority of transformation, which translated the unthinkable and was like the blueprint of a building opening, and in the impressive details he presented to us, we were constantly involved in interpreting everything he had heard from God.

During the time of the pandemic, also online, Dr. Don Lynch mentioned something about the seasons we live in that is worth a little reflection, sharing the care we need to take, focusing inherently on Christ and all his Word. On that occasion, he considered that we encounter three types of people:

1.	**The Confused**: The first figure are those people who are confused and can't discern what steps to take when faced with difficulties and circumstances beyond their control. An example we can all remember is in the old Tom and Jerry videos, when the little mouse would run around, knocking on every door he saw, trying to open them to escape the feline attack that wouldn't leave him alone for a second. This is how many people live, who, out of desperation in certain situations, look for alternatives without discerning which door they are knocking on to find their immediate satisfaction.

2.	**Comfort Seekers**: Secondly, we see people who need comfort, and who can or hope to be embraced and reached to feel better and more focused. And if you're that person who always needs another hug, seeking comfort and shelter from the affection of others, well, you're not alone, because you're where millions of others are. Often, they're in this place because they've done everything they can - or believe they can - only to find themselves, sadly, in positions of exhaustion and doubt, and ultimately, hopelessness. By the end of this book - if that person is you - you will understand that you are not alone in this battle. So don't give up pursuing the best in this journey and remember who is first in your life.

3.	**The Connected**: And the third figure has to do with those who recognize the times they live in, like the sons of Issachar, who act strategically and know the times they live in very well. (In my book *"When I Find Strength"*, I talk in more detail about the sons of Issachar.) Now, if you have been that connected person who knows the times, remember that everything you have received from God has come to you to be shared and reinvested, like a river that flows down the mountains and spreads out in trails that will provide enough for others to benefit from. It's like the parable of the sower who scatters seeds and, once sown, they will reach both the most confused and those who need a hug.

It doesn't matter where you are now. If your case is more like the first picture, you may be exactly where millions of post-pandemic people are. Some lost, confused, others challenged and unfocused on the next steps. We've noticed that malignancy has taken on a greater velocity and has thus come to blur the emotional lenses of people with less knowledge or a flawed relationship with God. However, even if people use their devices as an excuse, they will be pushed towards something greater and, ultimately, even without realizing it, they may also be part of this generation of knowers of the times. This is the power of God's Word in us and through us.

We have learned that if God is moving us into a new season, it would be very unwise to try to restore life to the way we lived before the coronavirus. These considerations serve as quick and necessary growth for those who serve the good Lord from the heart. This is a time to pay close attention to what the Bible tells us: "To live is Christ and to die is gain", and then to ask: "How much do I really believe this?". "Humble yourselves in the presence of the Lord, and he will exalt you.".[5]

"Blessed are the poor in spirit, for theirs is the kingdom of heaven. Blessed are those who mourn, for they will be comforted. Blessed are the meek, for they will inherit the earth. Blessed are those who hunger and thirst for righteousness, for they will be filled. Blessed are the merciful, for they will be shown mercy. Blessed are the pure in heart, for they will see God." [Mathew 5.3-8]

Necessary confrontation

Every change in mentality requires effort before you can understand and accept the confrontation of transformation. The body asks for the comfortable and, at the end of the day, the tendency is to say: *"I've done my bit"*. But what is this part that is still missing? The God First concept is designed to encourage people to leave their cozy little corner - their comfort zone - or that special area that only you know about, until it becomes a way of life. Reading about the 'God First' concept means entering the fray and allowing your mindset to be completely touched by curiosity, until your inspiration becomes sharp. Trying to live this content in a serious and distinctive way has never been easy and may become your greatest challenge until that day comes when you stand before your Heavenly Father. We're on this journey together!

In the confrontation of transformation, however, there is plenty of room for strategy and maturity. Just as you wouldn't feed a baby feijoada and solid food before its time, children in the faith must be respected before being put through challenging life moments. Maturity becomes more apparent when a person understands the extent of the responsibility they may experience. Not for this reason should the nourishing Word be rejected. If you are new to the faith and seek the truth with a sincere understanding and frankness, read, contextualize, reflect and pray; don't judge in advance.

If you want to learn faster, open the discussion with a Christian friend, find someone you trust, and argue about what you have read and learned. The Bible teaches that "by their fruits you will know them"! Talk, discuss, ask for guidance, talk to God and question every step that raises doubts. Also, don't hesitate to obey and act by faith. If you have any doubts, send me an e-mail and we can work together on this.

The reading of your fruits will always be evidenced by the results and compilations of this maturity acquired from many conversations, reading the Word and strategic meetings with the Holy Spirit. Try to live and socialize with authentic people - in addition to those who find it more difficult to be truthful, as we know, and who will always be present in our social groups. Our mission is to help them. Ask God and you will discover that there is something important here for your success in life.

The Importance of Awareness of the "God First" Lifestyle

It is essential to understand that the whole work of raising awareness of the "God First" lifestyle is intrinsically linked to individual faith. It's about being strong, even in moments of weakness, regardless of the circumstances. It's about doing what needs to be done and recognizing the transforming power that God exerts in the lives of those who stand on the truths of the Bible. This faith not only shapes character, but also allows a person to achieve great things, simply by believing and following the principles laid down by the Creator.

The Law of Sowing and Reaping

You've probably heard many stories of life transformation resulting from hard work, dedication to study or taking advantage of opportunities. This can be described as the Law of Sowing and Reaping: when someone invests hours of work, they will certainly reap the rewards of that effort. It is essential, however, to find a balance between what we have to do and the trust we place in Godl because here we are not only talking about achievements that are the result of human strength.

If, after much effort, the results are not what we expected, should we despair? Where is your declaration of faith and hope, knowing that God cares for us and is the provider of all who seek Him?

Salvation: A Gift

It's worth remembering that everyone can reap something they never planted: salvation. To do so, you must bow before the One who paid a high price and gave us the work of redemption. It's not something we earn; it's a gift that we don't deserve, but which has been given to us out of love.

In moments of challenge, we discover the depth of our statements of faith and the firm foundation of what we know and believe. Unfortunately, many religious circles are full of people who just repeat empty words, jargon and phrases that superficially touch the soul. In times of greatest need, these repetitions lead nowhere. The spirit is not fed, and this leads people away from biblical truth. When they should be resting in God, many plunge into despair, because they live in a shallow pool of experiences, with no room to go deeper.

No one can live off the ashes or the testimonies of others. It is crucial to experience something new every day. The experiences that God gives us generate maturity and activate the maintenance necessary for our lifestyle to be increasingly grounded and effective. This begins by opening our eyes every morning and talking to God. Throughout the day, we must listen to His voice, remembering that while we sleep or are awake, He takes care of every strategy necessary for our victory. Therefore, everything that happens in our lives must be investigated and reflected upon in the light of faith:

- "What is the purpose of this?".
- "How can I honor God in this matter?".
- "Was this an answer to prayer?".

Being transformed by purpose

When you get up, before your feet touch the floor of your room, ask: *"Father, how can I be used today?"*. Find your question - this is one of mine - and trust God first and foremost.

The season we live in expects, as always, that truths are not just read and spoken, but that they are demonstrated to the point of influencing and changing habits and customs that remove us from the presence of and communion with the Lord. Society squeezes believers to stifle them or to generate fruit, often from blind religiosity. We live in a time when the words echoed from pulpits are now seen and broadcast live by the media to every corner of the earth. Hence the great need for maturity that needs to be evident if the church - the person - really wants to influence society. The relevance of the relationship with God is demonstrated at every meeting, by the strategy of outreach and transformation, whether within homes or in the business market, but let the listeners be led to a purpose with God. Let true testimonies anchored in personal faith appear, based on their life examples.

Are you going to talk about Jesus? Then live your concepts!

Are you going to talk about the Word? Then get to know it as much as possible! This is the lifestyle expected in the Kingdom of God, in this heavenly government where we are commanded to multiply.

King David died centuries ago, yet to this day he is remembered as a great general by the Jews and by millions of people for an obvious reason: his testimony was the legacy he left to the generations. David took care of what had been placed in his hands, he received an anointing to be king and didn't lose sight of it, he was a battle general and a great conqueror. Above all, David became a worshipper in whom God greatly rejoiced. David wasn't perfect, but he was determined to do everything he needed to, in repentance and courage, honor his God.

Like David, God's beloved psalmist, you too must review your paradigms and perhaps change some of your apparent and supposed truths. It's up to you whether there will be room for change in this legacy that is your life, your God First lifestyle.

Ask yourself:

- What can the principles of Jesus and the Holy Spirit do to a person like me?
- What can the Word of God do on earth through me, if I live it faithfully?
- What would be the impact when the culture of the Kingdom implanted in me influences my environment outside the four walls of the church?
- What is my value to this generation?
- What legacy can I leave?
- How will I be remembered when I'm no longer here?

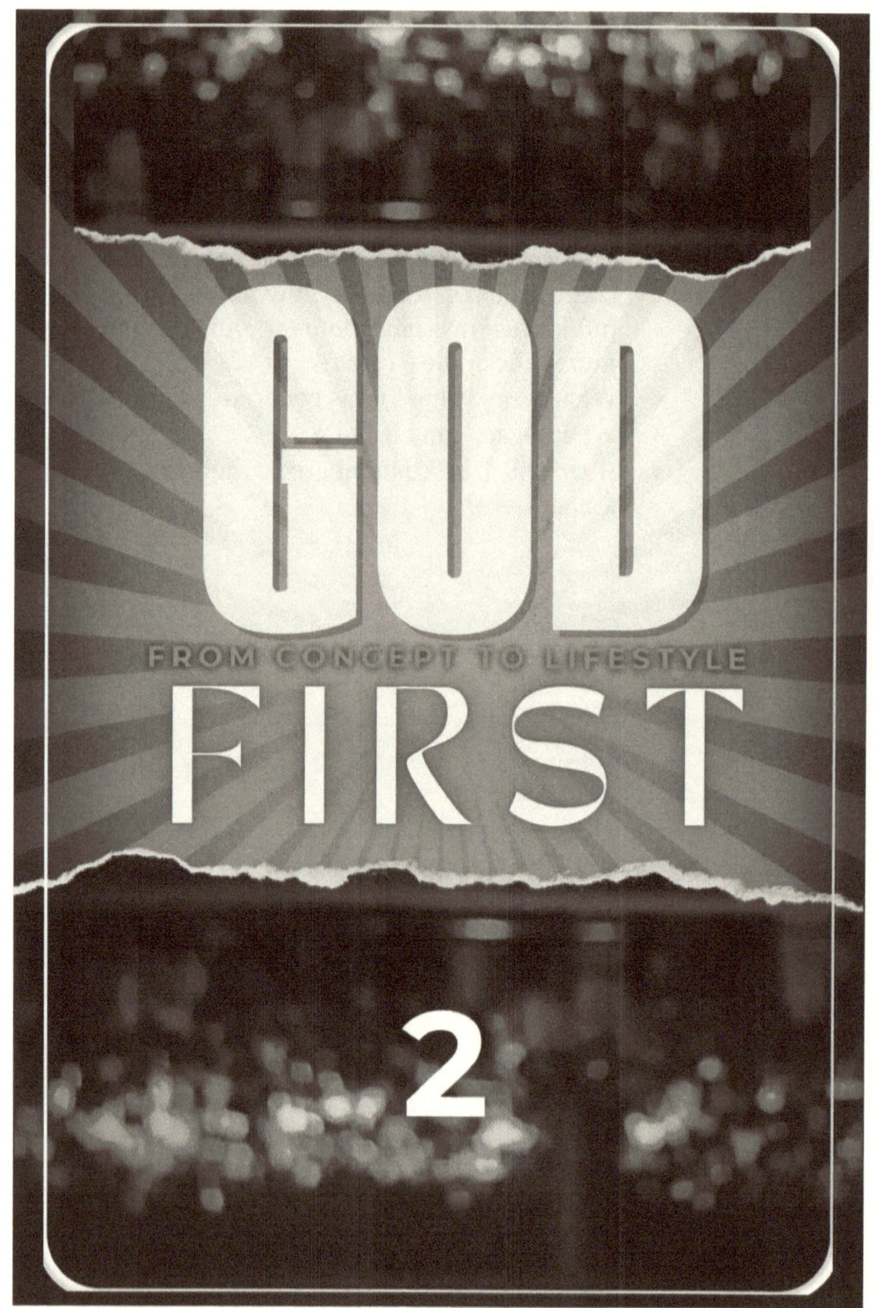

GOD
FROM CONCEPT TO LIFESTYLE
FIRST
2

2 - ONE MORE DEGREE

"We don't have to celebrate all growth. We celebrate the growth that's good!"

Teo Hayashi

The God First organization came about in a very unusual and curious way. For a few months, we met at home with about a dozen people. Everyone was very excited, and we couldn't wait for the moments of communion; every word shared, every invitation to change and transformation excited us. It wasn't a closed group; in fact, it was a gathering of friends who represented society in all its diversity. We had entreprencurs, musicians, lawyers, engineers, insurance salesmen, teachers and self-employed people, all with a great desire for inner change. We studied every detail of God's Word seriously.

During this same period, at the end of a journey of almost 20 days of ministering in various American states, I visited a church of friends who were completely involved in missionary work, Adilson and Marta Roberts. The two of them impressed me with the joy they conveyed and the fruit that the Holy Spirit had generated among them. It was at their home that I was able to enjoy a passion fruit juice with fruit picked right there in Florida, something not very common due to the climatic conditions of the region. But Pastor Adilson took on the challenge of pollination, and the result was a harvest with beautiful fruit and even better juice.

What a moment we had there, with the whole church worshipping and being prepared for the evangelization of Brazilians living in the surrounding small towns. The next day, my friends gave me a hardback book entitled *When God Is First*, by Mike Hayes. I was very grateful and went on my way to the airport.

Already on the plane, looking forward to returning home and seeing our Bible study friends again, I started reading the book and was deeply touched by the words that we now believe were inspired by the Holy Spirit. The words seemed to jump out at me. I was tremendously impacted by the message, and for hours I savored the valuable concepts written there. Pardon the pun, but the hours literally flew by. The plane landed and I happily arrived back in Brazil. Soon I was in the car, on my way home. Juliana and I talked about many things, but I couldn't leave out what had captured my attention while reading that book. Ju also started reading it and, like me, was struck by the seriousness of the message. You see, up until that moment, we hadn't decided on a name for what would become our future church.

A few days passed and, one afternoon, when we were almost home, Ju said: *"Could the name of our church be God First?"* Thoughtful but excited, we saw that the Word of God was right before our eyes as a confirmation. Yes, the name had caught on and was very fitting for the moment we were living in.

A simple concept, because in our hearts, and for most Christians, God must always be first. We decided to go one step further and seek to go beyond the concept, transforming it, possible, into a full reason and lifestyle.

When we were looking for more foundations from God for the study group we had just started, we came across the book of Isaiah, which reads:

> *"Thus says the Lord, the King of Israel, their Redeemer, the Lord of hosts: I am the first and I am the last, and besides me there is no God."* [Isaiah 44:6]

Even though it was just another verse establishing the lordship and greatness of God, Jesus, His Son and the wonderful presence of the Holy Spirit, God First, the text jumped out at us and, from that day on, we shared it with everyone, realizing that, in this triune form, we see that God is First, always has been and always will be! Want more?

> *"But seek first the kingdom of God and his righteousness, and all these things will be added to you."* [Mathew 6.33]

I believe that one of the main reasons we embarked on the mission of starting a study group, which later became a church and became a reference for many others, was the fact that we had a burning desire to share what was being built up in us. The desire not to keep and archive the seeds we received urged us not to give up and to be ever more persistent, looking ahead and always hoping for the best. We understood that the afflictions of the righteous are compensated for by God's mercy and love for everyone he created. The mission of God First today is:

"To redeem and conquer the earth through relevance and influence, representing and expanding Christ's Kingdom, His culture and salvation."

This desire to bring transformation to the society in which we live and to always be able to share what we have learned with our brothers and sisters from other denominations has always motivated us. I remember watching a documentary called *The Salt of the Earth*, where the photos and photographic experiences portrayed fallen humanity, human savagery and the tears that cannot be contained when one shows the degree of cynicism and hypocrisy of a person and how far a generation can go, inevitably wreaking emotional havoc on thousands of victims. Another side of this documentary, reflected in the passionate details of each photo, is the ability of the earth, through human care and work, to return to its original state, if we just do what we must. People and seasons can overthrow and destroy dreams, droughts come, wars are born, and indifference takes over everything; however, when we are ready to act, anything may be possible.

My goal, as a person, and our commitment, as children of God, has been to rebuild, because if nature is capable of this, we must observe its example and believe in what God expects and can do with us as well. It is the repetition of the transformative story in and through us. We can be this farmer, sculptor, restorer of souls. The final chapter in life that we will present will be the individual result of our actions; of how we will work with what seemed to have been destroyed.

The fall of man and its consequences

The fall of man, as described in Genesis 3:17-18, marks the moment when Adam and Eve disobeyed God by eating the forbidden fruit, being deceived by the devil and led into sin. As a result of this disobedience, God pronounced curses upon the earth and upon man's life. He warned Adam that the ground would be cursed because of him, and that man would have to work hard to obtain his sustenance, facing thorns and thistles. This passage symbolizes the introduction of suffering, hard work, and the separation between man and the fullness of life that God had originally planned for humanity.

It is important to note that we cannot assume that once man is morally reconstructed, all the world's problems will be solved. Therefore, in addition to striving to do our best, humanity's focus should be on looking to Christ, waiting for the moment when He comes to reign so that there may finally be complete restoration.

The reality of the human condition

Considering the malignancy exacerbated by man's declining moral condition, it is natural to think that God is not interested in protecting us, leading us to believe that we must fight alone to overcome difficulties. However, this view is misguided. We are reaping, as a society, what we have sown over the centuries. Since the world experienced this distancing from God, it has been cursed, and today society faces the consequences of this separation, seeking to solve, on its own, the problems that have arisen since then.

Humanity has failed to care for its own land, its people, and most importantly, for itself. My mission, as an individual responsibility, and what I seek as my part, is to move forward and make a difference by generating some transformation. This involves removing what has been wrongly instilled in me and in others, presenting the foundations that truly promote spiritual transformation. The wave I can generate may be small or perhaps larger than I ever imagined, but I am clear that it can at least take me to the next level of life.

Thus, the fall of man is not just an isolated event but a call to reflection and action. By recognizing the gravity of our separation from God and the need for transformation, we can seek a path that leads us to a fuller and more meaningful future, grounded in faith and hope in Christ. This journey requires us to take individual responsibility and work to promote the change we wish to see in the world.

For the truth, a choice to be made

I want to point here about the 10 lepers that Jesus ministered to. They were completely lost, forgotten and rejected by society. They felt abandoned. Until someone came along and gave them hope. Jesus broke the barrier of the impossible, of neglect, and proved that something could be done, regardless of what others thought or how culture had set its rules.

I often jokingly say to believers who don't attend their local church very often or to those who stop going to services for any other reason that is more important than being in the house of the Lord: "Are you from the God First church or the God is Second church?". At the end of the story, what seems to be a joke could be more serious than we think. If we want to live, to go one step higher, to be transformed and transformative to the point of becoming influential, God must be first in our hearts in any situation. This implies being honest with our inner reality, being real men and women, taking the risk of letting go of some pleasures to stop feeding our soul 'first'. Otherwise, we lie to ourselves and to the God who loved us first.

"Let us not forsake the assembling of ourselves together as a church, as the manner of some is; but let us encourage one another, all the more as you see the Day approaching." [Hebrews 10.25]

God chooses, separates, reserves, prepares and uses

One of our pastors, before he came to know Christ and much younger than me, was going through some difficult times in his life, being influenced by events of great sadness that he saw happening in his family and to dear friends. After accepting an invitation and taking part in our cell meetings, he fearlessly turned to God, believing in restoration and biblical guidance. Soon after, Wesley and Fabiana opened their home for Bible studies and dozens of people were able to come to know God, taking advantage of their influence and charisma. There was a lot of growth and Wesley was open to the options he read and heard. He sought answers from doctors and friends but discovered that the best option was to listen to the voice of the Holy Spirit in his life.

After some time and already knowing the Word, but still struggling with issues that troubled him, he took a piece of advice and decided to practice a sport more consistently. This would help him emotionally and increase the possibility of the healing he so desperately sought. He chose to do Jiu-Jitsu at a gym near his home, which helped him lower his anxiety. At the same time, he began to study the Word and, before long, he was no longer affected by his previously disturbing thoughts.

God always has a bigger plan!

One day, less than a year later, in a seemingly disinterested conversation, we concluded: we were going to combine Bible and sport to help other people. We decided to start a project in our city, Barueri (São Paulo, Brazil) to bring together young people from the periphery, mutual friends and whoever else wanted to, and help them practice the "gentle art" of Jiu-Jitsu with us - gentle in name only!

So, as he had been healed by God, we believed that others could also be reached, and the suggestion was accepted by everyone. But we had a problem: who would be the teacher? We prayed and one day, while we were gathered with some families for an end-of-year dinner, something happened. Just as Jeremiah heard the voice of the Lord, it was as if *"the word of the Lord came to me"*. There was a labor judge there, a black belt, who trained at the same gym as us and the first chance I got, I asked him: *"Would you like to join us and teach the people we're going to invite to a social project in our space?"* He immediately accepted.

That spurred us on, and we worked on the details to get the project off the ground. In the same week, another teacher joined, our friend Bercê, who already took part in our meetings. We saw the movement of God's plan, who used us as instruments for something greater to happen.

Our mission to redeem and win people for the kingdom through relevance and influence is in full swing. At every training session, we pray with the athletes and give a devotional. Since 1915, hundreds of people have been trained, state and national champions have come out of the project, and we have fallen in love with sport. Many people and events have helped us to solidify the project, which has now been consolidated as an *NGO - DP Transforma* - and we are honored to serve the Lord with a focus on rescuing and transforming lives for the kingdom of God.

It could well be your starting point to do missions in Brazil.

Here comes Samurai!

Recently, a whole family started training with us, and the difference is that Mathias, Leandro and Roberta's son, became our mascot. Diagnosed with autism, Mathias subtly showed signs of the condition, which initially made us think it would be a challenge for him. Jiu-Jitsu is a sport that requires grappling and uses every move as if it were a chess move, involving constant physical contact. However, Mathias accepted the challenge and left us impressed with his tenacity and dedication to the sport.

For those who have no experience of autism and are unaware of the different degrees that diagnosed people face, Mathias' performance was a pleasant surprise. He stood out as an excellent student and taught us that, regardless of the diagnosis, everyone can learn and grow. Our dear Mathias, affectionately called "Samurai", demonstrates how God cares for and blesses those who seek him.

In addition to his performance on the mat, we enjoy Mathias' genius in other areas. If anyone has any doubts about the history of trains around the world or questions about world geography, just ask him; he knows all about locomotives and flags - and answers immediately. It's impressive how Jiu-Jitsu not only promotes social inclusion, but also offers significant benefits for children with Autism Spectrum Disorder (ASD), such as improved motor coordination, social interaction and emotional development.

The relevance of the project

In one of our meetings off the mat, I remember saying to the Judge, who is also known as Lobo: *"I just wanted to tell you that, before you hear it from anyone else, I've been using your example to illustrate how God works in people's hearts and accomplishes His purposes. When we opened this project, what encouraged us most was the possibility of bringing the person of Christ to your heart!"* As I was speaking, I was interrupted; he stood up and declared incisively: *"Marcos, sorry for the interruption, but I just wanted to say that you have already achieved this purpose!"* We laughed a lot, but it was a laugh of joy at realizing that many of the objectives that motivated us to start the project have been achieved.

These testimonies, among the many we have already shared, show how God connects the dots, people and our wills to achieve lasting purposes. All of this serves as a response to the lifestyle we seek to share and has happened because, one day, we decided to listen to the voice of the Holy Spirit and take active action.

Being relevant in society means being aware of your role and focusing primarily on winning someone to Christ. With this message, we can become agents of transformation in a new lifestyle.

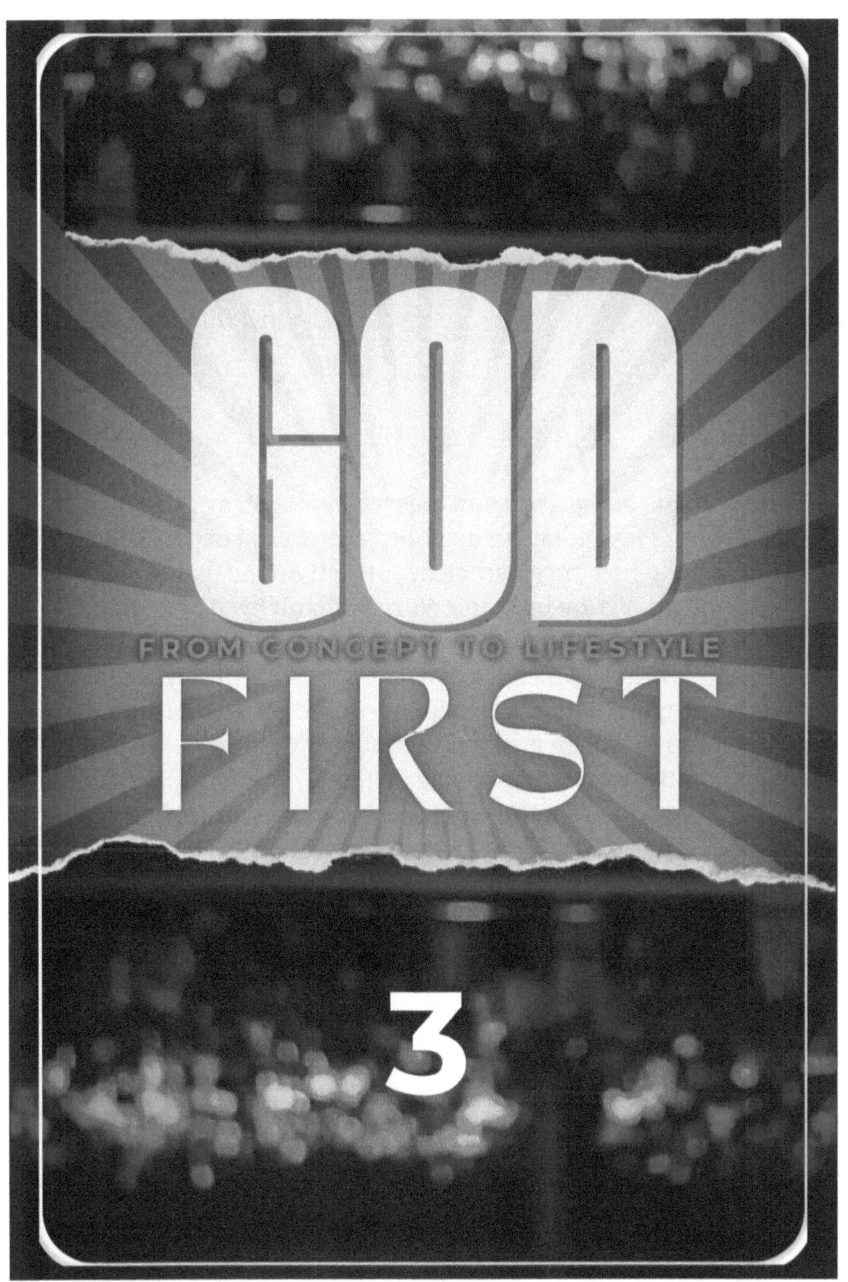

GOD
FROM CONCEPT TO LIFESTYLE
FIRST
3

It's not enough to have good thoughts. We need to have the courage to defend them."

Albus Dumbledore

One of the great and blessed points of my growth is the joy of having been born into a Christian home, where I received clear, objective and panoramic instruction from the Word which, if lived according to what is laid down, makes all the difference in the world in which we live. The secret to this joy is that my parents never taught me and my two brothers to live in an evangelical bubble. My experience has always been studying, playing or working with people from the most diverse beliefs and religions.

Even without much knowledge, but accepting the challenges I faced, my heart was almost always focused on discovering the power of Jesus that was proclaimed in my home and by my Sunday Morning teachers. In this way, I was always curious and observed the paths and results that were generated by people inside and outside the churches. I've seen people who were born into homes with Christian parents and learned biblical principles from childhood; I've walked with friends who met Jesus halfway and clung to the truth in search of genuine transformation; and I've seen people who never had the opportunity to have Christian parents and weren't taught the principles and lenses of the Gospel that lead a person to know themselves better. The results are so widespread in society that we are amazed. ***Someone who changes their values in exchange for interests has never had value!"***

Even if you fit into one of the above options, you may have already discovered that nothing happens simply and automatically. When a person decides to live according to the Gospel of Christ, they stop being mere creatures of God and start living as His children. On their journey, they learn and discover the need to change certain paradigms that have been generated in family or religious tradition. Every relationship or character of a person reflects the result of a process of reconstruction or destruction, based on the choices they have made and are making.

At a certain point in life, each person will be exposed to new concepts that can be challenging and, in this process - of checking whether their choices were right or wrong - they may find it difficult to believe or accept the change in concepts that, for many years, have been orchestrated and sealed inside them as a manipulation of the soul. This difficulty may stem from experiences and learning within the home, from religiosity or pride and, as is the case with most people, from the fear of experiencing the new.

Life's challenges

It's interesting to think that having attended church since I was a child, I've always considered myself saved, enjoying the promised inheritance - which really is a great gift - of having believing parents who knew how to teach the principles on which I'm established as an adult to this day.

However, this is no guarantee of a sinless life. For me, however, apart from the wonderful fact of growing up away from the evil and teachings that keep us from this inheritance, I also understand that there is a danger that is not always perceived, which can easily deceive us. Being in the church or being a member of it does not qualify anyone as a child of God! Being called a child implies a full surrender of spirit, soul and body to the mission we receive when we give ourselves up. Then it's about being in the church, being a member and learning the strategies at its headquarters.

The deception that many people experience, just as I did, believing that nothing was wrong with my lifestyle, can be the factor that causes a lot of damage to the entire evangelical system. My keen - and at the time, not very positive - critical sense of people who weren't like me, believers and churchgoers, further built up who I didn't need to become. I made a departmentalization of everything around me: believer's stuff, world stuff; sacred music, profane music; long hair, short hair; play ball, don't play ball; speak in tongues, don't speak in tongues... Inadvertently, I was part of the statistics, adding up to millions of Christians, but I was religious in the way I lived.

Self-knowledge and others!

I criticized the more traditional denominations for not being open to the manifestations of the Holy Spirit; I criticized the way the more Pentecostal ones dressed and manifested themselves; I observed everything and everyone. I also saw that my friends and I weren't the only ones living like this. We discovered that our religious lifestyle was just another facet that we had learned from the generation before us. We looked outwards and at others, but little at our own inner self and relationship with God. And, just as in Jesus' time, when his criticism was used to show up the atrocities taught by the Pharisees, we have seen that the religious system is still active and operating, taking away people's option to live without the politicking that we witness in places where we set foot, and which many call church.

Incredibly, I studied and read the Bible, walked in character and was respected for it; I was happy because I was recognized as someone who always sought to do what was right and respectful. Even so, the Christian jargon, many manias, words and attitudes that could and should be corrected, were left to one side, because everyone around me did it that way. How could this happen?

Did you know that religiosity can take you to a dimension far removed from that expected and announced by Jesus? It can quietly and subtly remove us from the Kingdom of God and transport us to another place, the Kingdom of Secularism, because that's exactly how the devil works.

> *"This question was only raised because of some false brothers who infiltrated our midst to spy on us and take away the freedom we have in Christ Jesus. Their intention was to enslave us..."* [Galatians 2:4].

Attention!

Do you seek God and want Him to always be first in everything you do? Very good, but it's time to open our eyes, because often we think we are so used and needed in the Lord's work that a lack of zeal gives us away. The exercise to get out of this place of deception is to investigate yourself as soon as possible, get to know yourself better and develop a keen self-knowledge. The fact is that we have accumulated characteristics that are neither welcome nor in keeping with the truth. That's why they shouldn't be part of our pattern of behavior. The *"false brothers"* that the apostle Paul commented on above certainly lived among the people in the congregations he taught, influencing, talking to and exchanging experiences all the time, but in fact they were not followers of Christ or did not understand the fullness of the good news.

It's one thing to be born and raised on the best principles within your home or from the moment you give yourself to the Lord. It's quite another to live them to the full. In the religiosity that is so common among all of us, the good and blessing principles are set aside, which are so often justified by the fact that we attend services, sing, give offerings, tithe and evangelize others; and all of this is good. But what kind of multiplication are we promoting if we still want performance and depend on what others think of us?

It's sad to think that this is the basis that many use and aspire in order to rise and have eternal life with the Lord. You've seen singers, evangelists, pastors and members falling into disgrace, doing all the things I mentioned above. What's worse, today we're watching many of them fall live in the media or online. And, with this increasing every day and people far from a life surrendered to God, added to the bad example of life that many give and reproduce inside and outside their homes, a weak and unhealthy generation is consistently developing.

Meek as a dove, cunning as a serpent

You've seen this movie before. Someone famous starts attending meetings and people are intimidated for fear of the repercussions or that they will stop congregating with everyone - because the famous bring media, don't they? But who says that the rules and principles of the old paths can be changed to suit someone with greater repercussions? This is fighting against what the Bible says. We have put people on the altar where God should be, no matter how important they are. The focus and the stage must always be God First.

A few years ago, we had a very famous person who attended our weekly services. At first, my mind said: *"I'll leave her there, out of focus, until she grows in the Word"*. The thought was right. I checked with other pastor friends and one of them told me: *"Some people are going to reach hundreds of people, other millions of people"*. Months passed and, as much as we sought to call her to a growth and relationship with God, nothing deeper happened.

What do people want today? Whether they're famous or not, they're looking for a place where they'll be accepted, if they don't have to change. And this has been a problem that doesn't just affect influential personalities. Parents are looking for a place where their children will be liked and cared for, and not where God often wants them to grow healthily as a family.

Excuses pile up and, if expectations are low, no church will ever be good enough. That famous person couldn't stand it and gave up on God, no matter how dear they were, they couldn't stand the test that the Gospel demands of each person. Before long, her family was torn apart by divorce and her faith, being tested, didn't hold up and she gave in to the demands of the world without God. But she is still remembered in our prayer times because we love her. Jesus warned us that each person must carry their own cross.

Persistence, patience and results

Life with God requires transformation, and this doesn't happen without persistence and care. Even though I lived surrounded by the Word that set me free, it wasn't until I was eighteen that I made the personal decision to follow Christ. I didn't accept Him because of illness or lack of options; I didn't accept Him just because my parents were believers and gave me good examples; I didn't accept Him because my soccer friends were also in the church. I was in one of the best phases of my life: emotionally, spiritually and financially. But at one of the Sunday morning services, sitting comfortably in the back pews, where my friends and I usually met, it was there that I surrendered, talking to God, quiet in my spirit, but humbly listening to what He had to say. Suddenly, I was no longer there just to see my friends again. I wasn't there to satisfy my parents.

I was fine, and that day my life changed radically. Jesus came like a tsunami into my being, changed everything and restructured my interior. From that split second, a gradual demolition of structures that had been built and formed over time began. I needed friends, my parents, my leaders and a consistent reading of the Word so that I could discover what I had always been looking for and hadn't found until then. And it was from that day on that my foundation in life was restored. Many years have passed and, up to this point in my life, I know that there is still room for change.

One of the first realizations that came to me was that there was no separation between being a believer inside or outside the church. I remembered when Jesus called the disciples, one by one, using what they did best. I became aware that we are part of this earth to govern and establish something that the world has not yet seen in its fullness. I became aware that I am also responsible for establishing what the world has always sought and not found: peace in people's hearts. But all that would happen was what I heard from the Lord: that it would be a consistent and lasting process.

Even so, with so many expectations on my horizon, there were many moments when I thought it was all going to shit and I felt like I was fighting against something that often seemed like fiction. I had everything an 18-year-old would hope for: a supportive family, university, a job, friends, a car. However, at that beginning of the process, I was still the one who ran my life and I clearly behaved like everyone else in unbelieving society, that is, I led my life without God being at the center of it, without Him being First in everything. The adjustment that the Holy Spirit was asking of me required correcting paths that I didn't even know existed. From that morning on, my desires, my dreams, my wishes, my goals, everything went through the sieve, and I was willing because I felt God's voice, and I wanted to change. Consciously, I removed myself from the chair of control that I had comfortably occupied for longer than I should have and gave God space, allowing Him to take over.

In truth, there was an internal struggle, because my soul wasn't ready for what I was proposing, but it lost! In that very special moment, it was as if I saw a very large sign on the road, a billboard that reminded me: "Christ is not fiction"! I saw with joy that He is the only option for a full life, and I pressed the accelerator.

I discovered, being consistent in my position as an active member of the church, that the Holy Spirit, in His time and with the necessary space, takes charge of the journey and, from a new perspective, offers every help so that we can look at the reality of things as they really are, with experiences and responses of His working in everything we do and produce. In that season of change, it was very important for me to understand that, by reading the Word, there are facets of God that are there, ready to be revealed. He creates, gives life and transforms when we allow ourselves to be used by Him.

A lot of time has passed since that experience. I've stepped on the four corners of this earth and had the privilege of translating and living with dozens of great men and women; I've developed great relationships of friendship with many of these people and I've seen, learning from all of this, that the unique message that makes someone convinced and converted to Christ is primarily based on the way we live and are inside and outside the church. I discovered that true friends develop their communication of character even more when they are not seen by people. Discover for yourself that, alone or in a group, the gentle scent of the Holy Spirit is what will eventually convince anyone, but this scent needs to be exhaled through your life. And, of course, sometimes the results for the multiplication of God's kingdom come without any words, but through a shared lifestyle.

Fruit that remains

During their maturing process, people go through similar experiences, although their stories and choices vary. When I lived in São Paulo, I attended several Full Gospel meetings and met many businessmen, entrepreneurs, doctors, who came there with some hope of seeing things change. How many times I heard moving testimonies that helped each person in their process of transformation.

One evening, the speaker was Tony Portigliatti. He told moving stories of his initial process of restoration. He said: *"I was a business owner, I had my factory and distribution company, but when I accepted Jesus, the first thing that happened to me was bankruptcy."* Everyone laughed and at the same time embraced him with looks of respect and empathy. But he showed that he knew himself and had the courage to calmly recount his process. Yes, he went bankrupt, and he showed us that, for his story, everything he had been through was necessary for him to be able to rethink and rebuild an entire successful life.

It's not God's rule to make people go bankrupt when they accept Him, but He acts in whatever way He deems necessary until someone can get to where they need to be to walk within God's will. God specializes in showing us that the basis is Him, not man and his ability, and it is up to the person to identify with this facet of the Creator. That's why, on many occasions, we are repositioned on the first step so that, some time later, we can look back and give thanks for the process we have endured.

In the case of Tony, one of the most generous people I've ever met, he had the charisma, the ability, the love for souls and, even so, a lot of faith, decision and attitude had to be leveraged for his test on the path to give the result he has obtained. After many years of faith and persistence, as well as dozens of completed ventures, Dr. Portigliatti carries a legacy of being the creator of the process of ascension that Florida Christian University represents for thousands of students around the world. The culture and society he touches are influenced by this transformative spectrum and benefit from the students who are placed on the job market each semester. With his direct speech, he inspires us with the drive and boldness of someone who has seen things happen and strategic connections made.

Tony is a born entrepreneur, but for those of us who know him, he's not just a businessman, he's an ambassador for the Gospel, who leads a restored and prosperous life, actively fighting for his generation to continue the legacy. All that has happened has not come with the power of a magic wand, nor has it been by mere coincidence; there has certainly been a process of obedience, persistence and commitment in which, I believe, he does not regret the fruits that are out there. God has been first in his life.

> *"Search me, O God, and know my heart; try me and see my thoughts. Show me if there is anything in me that offends you, and lead me in the way everlasting."* [Psalm 139.23-24]

In this way, we see God putting together puzzles which, step by step, reveal humanity's paths to success. I'm bringing you stories that I've lived and seen in many people and, of course, we don't know all the details, nor the circumstances or the price that each person pays to get where they are. The difference for purposes to be fulfilled and targets to be achieved lies in developing a clear and objective Christian conscience so that, when called upon, everyone can be ready to respond immediately: *"I'm going, Lord!"*.

The reality of life is that no dream or step towards God is easy to achieve. Humanity muddles through the world, looking for complicated alternatives that are far removed from what is really needed to meet the Lord. The Bible doesn't require self-flagellation, animal sacrifices - let alone people - or any other means other than the one Jesus has already established in His Word. In my case, it all started with the search and intercession of my parents, who were always faithful to their calling and gave me the teaching and good examples I needed.

One generation transfers the best it has to the next, even with its human limitations. Even so, when I found myself faced with the many situations and circumstances that life presents, I had to readjust my course and allow myself to see God at work in all areas of my life, reluctantly at times. I had to find courage and boldness, humility and discipline - the latter being my greatest initial difficulty.

Without giving up and learning at every stage of life, we realize more and more that God wants to keep us on our toes, focusing our attention on the prize we hope to win. It's not best to come to God out of fear, the dread of death, uncertainty or the dozens of other questions that torment the heart. It is better to go through the process, whatever it may be.

Obviously, we don't expect people to seek God only because they are afraid of death or because they are sick and in need of healing. We think so, but for the One who waits for us with open arms, any time or situation is the right time to come to Him. God is the God of miracles and, at some point in our lives, we will long to be in that place of worship. It gives us abundant peace and makes us curious every morning. He will always be worshipped, and we will always have something to accomplish to establish God's kingdom.

"I'm not saying that I've already achieved all this, that I've already reached perfection. But I press on to conquer that perfection for which Christ Jesus conquered me. No, brethren, I have not attained it, but I focus all my efforts on this: forgetting the past and looking to what lies ahead, I press on to the finish of the race, to receive the heavenly prize for which God has called us in Christ Jesus." [Philippians 3.12-14]

You may be that person who is doing well financially, who has overcome personal struggles and has established yourself by reading good books, taking advice from honest people and perhaps you have made your commitment to a church and are actively part of it. Congratulations! It could be someone who has already found their routine of success and blessings, discovered in the Word the secret of a healthy relationship and, as well as being very successful in their profession, is also bold enough to pass on what has happened to them to others. This is exactly our role to fulfill, it's what should happen to the people who come to God in our worship services. My calling is to take even this kind of person to a new and higher level of understanding and commitment to God.

Look at what God does

Sérgio, a friend of many years, another dear friend with whom I had the pleasure of walking and even celebrating the birth of his first child, has always shown what he's made of in the business world. His tenacity and charisma make him a brilliant developer of ideas, and, for a long time, he was the manager of a multinational food company in Brazil. At the same time, during his maturing process, an unexpected blow came! From one day to the next, he found himself without the security of his position at work, and his financial fortunes would undoubtedly suffer a major blow. As a result, he spent a few years draining his savings and, no matter how hard he looked, the doors wouldn't open for him to fit back into the market. His thoughts struggled with his foundation of faith. Rejection, incapacity, despair, bankruptcy, all came to the surface, like a waterfall hitting his emotional base hard. Even though he was shaken at times, like a boxer, Sérgio would get up and show his family that he believed in something greater.

In reality, and we can understand this better today, God was preparing a divine strategy that would soon be put into action. If God's plan was not realized, there was crying, misunderstanding, embarrassment, etc. Even so, within him, a Christian awareness and spiritual growth were generated that made him unshakeable. With frequent disappointments in his attempts, his family didn't give up and remained faithful. The impediment to new challenges was not age, but quite possibly the need for them to discover their calling and vocation. In this process of searching for a place in the market, he discovered that he had never given himself so strongly to the truths of Jesus.

He also discovered that his search was greater and lighter when he first placed his greatest cries and questions in God. At the end of the tunnel, the light appeared. God gave him favor, creative ideas and friends. Remember that God is creator, He gives life and transforms. Years passed, and my friend's faith was tested, but the fruits were counted in his favor. His calling is to the business sphere, and Sérgio is the kind of person that no one can hold inside a church and say: "stay there!" Even so, because he has never stopped learning, he has always been a great friend and servant within the church we serve together.

We're talking about God First, the lifestyle that brings results, first for God's kingdom, but which increases our barns much more than if we had only focused on our own designs. Make no mistake here. Sérgio has always faithfully served his local church. Wherever his feet touch, charismatic that he is, he is not ashamed of his faith. Did he have to go through the school of maturity? Yes, we all must go through it and be approved. Each step taken is necessary, but it will lead us to where God wants us to be.

In every experience your children go through, God will always be present, whether it's the simplest or the most difficult. Our coach, Jesus and His Word, will support us until we can count success. Glory be to God for the experiences we must "face and for our insistence on not giving up until the end.

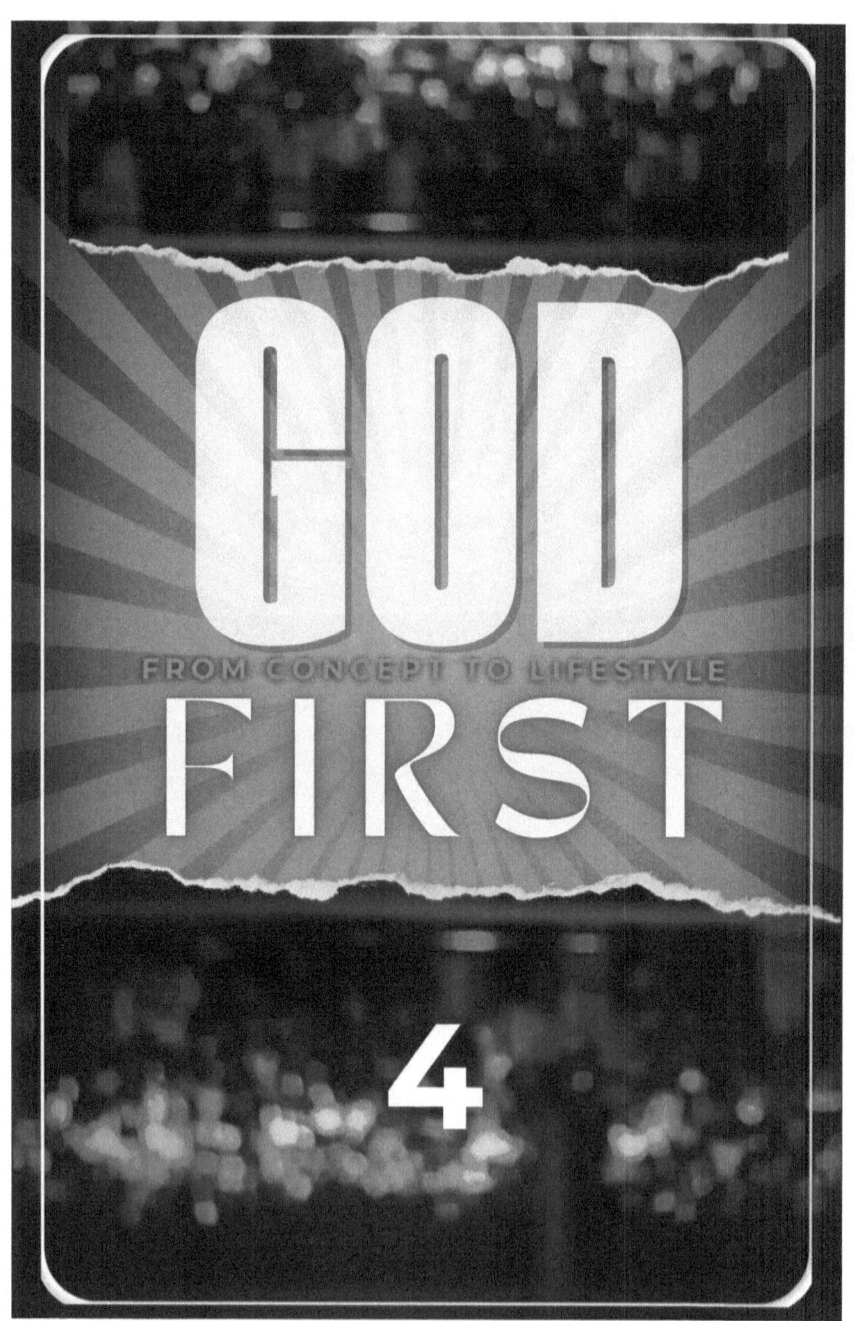

GOD
FROM CONCEPT TO LIFESTYLE
FIRST
4

4 - FROM ACHAN TO GEHAZI IN EACH ONE OF US! HOW TO GET OUT OF THIS.

"The heart is more deceitful than anything else and its disease is incurable. Who can understand it? "I am the Lord who searches the heart and examines the mind, to reward everyone according to his conduct, according to his deeds." [Jeremiah 17:9-10]

We are a living reflection of our choices! Just a glance in the rearview mirror of the past and I'm immediately reminded of the decisions I've made that have shaped the outcomes of the things I experience today. God's Word dives deep into these issues and presents me with powerful examples that lead me to a deeper contemplation of what I choose to do at every crossroads in life.

I focus my gaze on the children of Israel, who endured four centuries of slavery and another 40 years of hard walking in the desert as a direct consequence of their choices. The time had finally come when they would be established as a nation and God would give them a new name, just as he had done with Jacob. And, of course, more crucial choices had to be made.

Until then, the Israelites had only been known as "Hebrew slaves" or "Bedouins". But history was being shaped by the Spirit of the Lord, who was offering them a choice that would become the key to a glorious entry into the promised land. God demanded a commitment of great importance, which would serve as a compass for the rest of Israel's journey: that they be obedient and faithfully observe God's laws. Only by fulfilling this condition could the nation regain its authority before the nations and be known and approved as "the children of the one true God".

Of course, all this would be accompanied by all the blessings that God's name itself carries. The plan went into action; YHWH would be the top priority and the First in the whole nation. This commitment, however, would be evidenced by the authority of God's name and the incredible favor they would receive for acknowledging Him as Lord. Now history was taking a different turn, and Israel's enemies trembled at the name of the Israelites, "children of the one God", such was the favor and authority they demonstrated in this relationship of obedience!

Joshua, although initially reluctant because he didn't think he was up to the task, was chosen as the leader who would ignite the people to listen and follow God's voice with passion. Already near Jericho, while they were gathered and camped around the city, Joshua and the people of Israel were anxiously awaiting instructions to move on. The news of their presence in the fields surrounding the city was already known inside Jericho; there was disquiet, and fear was palpable among the enemies, which added to the terror among the residents of the city who, frightened, closed the gates and reinforced the walls of Jericho.

> "Now Jericho was shut up tightly because of the children of Israel; no one went out or came in." [Joshua 6.1]

Joshua warned, reminding the army of the Lord, that Jericho would be the first city to be conquered; that their choice would not be in vain, and was therefore the sign that other spectacular victories were to come, and everyone rejoiced. The instructions and details of the battle were passed on - by the Lord of the battle himself - and, with great reverential awe, they attended, for God had finally revealed the impressive plan of how he would give them the city.

We're talking about a war, but here, in the first city to be conquered, God said he would fight that battle for them, and no one would need to lift a sword. Humanly speaking, it seemed like a crazy plan, but we saw God surprisingly getting involved and once again demonstrating His supernatural care. But a crucial requirement loomed, and He - the One God - expected total obedience from all the people, and the proof of that faithfulness was yet to come. What we saw next you probably already know: Israel marched around Jericho once a day for six days and, on the seventh day, seven times. Then they shouted in unison, and the walls of Jericho came crashing down into the city.

Know one thing! Everything that comes from God for His loved ones, just like a simple flower in the field, blossoms and opens to glorious new prospects. And on the other hand, everything that revolts against or resists what has already been established for us will implode, because the enemy's plans will always be thwarted in the face of spiritual and heavenly action on behalf of the children. Yes, the walls of Jericho fell - imploded - into the city, in a resounding defeat!

Don't touch what God has consecrated!

Once conquered, it remained for God's people to take God's instruction seriously: don't touch anything inside the city and set fire to everything, because Jericho was "doomed to destruction". This command was not just a whim; God was conveying a lesson that still resonates today. In the original language, the word "doomed" is the same word from which we derive the term "consecrated". In some translations, we find the expression "consecrated for destruction". For Israel, this understanding was nothing new; everyone was very familiar with this concept, which was part of their worship rituals. The Lord wanted to make it clear that the first conquered city did not belong to them, nor did the wealth of that place.

Jericho had become an object of consecration and, at the same time, of destruction. And if God had warned them, they had better obey him!

When the city was destroyed, God's people were filled with faith! It was the first conquest, and all the gold and silver coins on display shone, symbolizing Jericho's riches. However, the order was clear: not to touch anything for themselves. The gold and silver were to be taken exclusively for the construction of the temple, nothing else. The people, still amazed at what God had done, rejoiced in their victory and believed in God's promise. Israel celebrated and saw that their choice had been approved. But in the spiritual world, something else was about to be revealed.

Just as our faith is tested every day by the choices we make, Achan's faith and obedience were exposed because he dared to disobey God's direct orders. While the people were sacking the city, gathering the tools for destruction and preparing to burn everything as an offering to the Lord, Achan's soul spoke louder. He couldn't resist what his heart desired, and greed took over. Taking advantage of the festive occasion, Achan decided to gather up his "discovery", camouflaged his "treasure" and headed for his tent. That same day, he dug a hole and buried his theft there.

How did Achan's conscience feel knowing that he was sinning? Something was clearly wrong, and he didn't celebrate it, he didn't share it with his fighting friends or even his family, because he knew it wouldn't be approved. It was his choice not to obey what God had presented as a crucial condition after the victory. In his heart, Achan decided to follow the pattern of war, which was to divide the spoils of battle among the soldiers. But this time, there was a higher order, which sought to transform man's pattern and lifestyle to build God's will. This would only happen if God was put first in the hearts of His children.

Still oblivious to what had happened in Achan's tent, Joshua and his soldiers were thrilled with the outcome and soon set off boldly towards what they hoped would be their second conquest. But the unexpected happened. The disappointment and embarrassment at the defeat in the city of Ai, seeing his men die, was only really understood when the Lord's words revealed the offense. The expected victory at Ai collapsed because something inexplicable was hovering in the spiritual atmosphere, where real things happen, and we often don't even notice. The answer was direct, and God's voice echoed so that there could be no doubt: "Israel has sinned and stolen my glory!"

One thing is certain, and we always learn this from the Bible: no one touches God's glory! The end was tragic, not just for Achan; his family also suffered the consequences of his unfaithfulness and were completely wiped off the earth. Read the book of Joshua carefully from the beginning to understand all this very important context.

Man will always have choices to make. Choices that can lead to blessing and multiplication or choices that can generate destructive consequences for his entire existence.

The prophet's servant

In the book of 2 Kings, we delve into another fascinating story that reveals man's difficulty in keeping his heart aligned with God. Once again, we can clearly see the results of the choices we make. Naaman, a war hero and commander of the Syrian king's army, was seriously ill. His body was taken over by leprosy, a terrible and incurable disease. But then his servant intervened with an inspired suggestion: if he could stand before the prophet in Samaria, he could be restored from leprosy. Impressive is the value of this slave girl's testimony and her unwavering trust in her God, even though she was far from her homeland. Naaman accepted the advice and didn't give up until he reached the door of Elisha's house.

First, the commander did what every good soldier should do: he asked the king for permission to go on his way and went out focused on the result he hoped to achieve. He obeyed the process. Naaman, believing in formality, went straight to the king of Israel, who was at a loss as to what to do. From there, he was sent to the prophet Elisha. Elisha, for his part, knew that many prophets spoke more than they should and did less than they needed to. So, he sent a message to the king:

"Send Naaman to me, and he will know that there is a true prophet in Israel." [2Kings 5.8]

Even though he knew who the commander was, Elisha asked Gehazi to instruct Naaman to wash in the river Jordan seven times and his skin would be restored. Naaman, most likely shocked and surprised to see his authority ignored, had his first shock of reality and became indignant. It seemed that the prophet had not received him with the honors he deserved. He looked at natural things, compared the beautiful rivers of his land and felt humiliated at having to do something he didn't think was appropriate.

Once again, Naaman was helped by people the Bible doesn't even mention by name: first, the slave "girl", and now, his own "officials" advised him to obey. But Naaman, a disciplined and dutiful soldier, obediently went ahead and was completely healed.

"So Naaman went down to the Jordan and dipped seven times, as instructed by the man of God. His skin became as healthy as a child's, and he was healed." [2 Kings 5.14]

After this, Naaman returned with his entire entourage and went to meet the man of God, bringing valuable gifts to repay the favor. The commander recognized the power of the one who had healed him and declared: "Now I know that there is no God in all the world but in Israel" [2Kgs 5.15]. Elisha chose to refuse the gifts, preferring to give all the glory to God. Naaman, still grateful, came away understanding the true worship that should be given to the God who healed him. He promised not to serve other gods anymore, only the Lord.

But Gehazi, Elisha's servant

But then someone comes on the scene again, with the intention of taking advantage of something that didn't belong to him:

> " Gehazi, the servant of Elisha the man of God, said to himself, 'My master was too easy on Naaman, this Aramean, by not accepting from him what he brought. As surely as the Lord lives, I will run after him and get something from him.'" [2 kings 5.20]

There is a voice that constantly speaks in people's ears, whether they are leaders, men or women, religious or not; a voice that, after evaluating a situation, asks if "this" is right, "if I haven't lost anything with this", or "what will be left for me?". This is the voice of conscience. If there are weaknesses, this voice takes advantage of the situation and instigates the person's soul to negotiate with the wrong or evil that is stored somewhere inside, deep in their heart, just waiting for the opportune moment to strike.

Gehazi thought! He wished! He chose and used God's name to justify himself! And, as we saw earlier with Achan, who went after what he imagined to be his "opportunity" for success, Gehazi also succumbed.

Gehazi hurried, stopped Naaman's entourage, lied and sought to take advantage of what his master had chosen to avoid. The prophet didn't want to receive gifts to give all the glory to God and set an example to someone who had just experienced healing. Gehazi didn't reflect on these aspects, and his heart was only set on gain, even if it was clearly undue and unfair.

The whole strategy set up in his thoughts for a human conquest blinded him and closed his spirit and soul to the peace of God. With that attitude, Gehazi also blocked his own path to so many other blessings that would have been in his hands as a helper to someone who honored his calling.

Bringing this to our day, Gehazi can represent the "good boy", the correct believer, the one who has opportunities to walk with men of God, to attend conferences and participate in powerful and popular ministries. Or he could be the man of God himself who, as well as observing and seeing great miracles taking place, is already doing very well in his field of ministry. Even so, he decides to commit himself to "the king's delicacies" of the world of opportunities and chooses not to observe the victories of the Spirit and decides that his ideas are better and don't even need to be questioned before they are put into effect.

Gehazi, who saw and enjoyed the company of the prophet, witnessed tremendous miracles and even took part in some of them, as in the case of the woman who saw her son die, but who, through the power of God and the interference of both Gehazi and the prophet, saw the miracle of her son's resurrection. Even so, the opportunity that so many others wanted to have, and that God had given her, was not used properly.

If you continue reading 2 Kings, you'll notice that Gehazi lied not only in the name of God, but also in the name of the prophet. And to a certain extent, he seemed to believe he was doing the right thing. That's how it is with many people, unfortunately. They do the wrong thing and justify themselves by lying, presenting themselves as serious men of God, placing themselves as holy and blameless before the Father, as if God would accept them unconditionally. Everything that happens in the natural and we think is hidden, is certainly revealed in the spiritual, where accounts are settled and decided. Don't forget that we have an eternal Advocate and Judge. Here is the outcome of this story:

> *"But he went in and stood before his master. Elisha said to him, 'Where are you coming from, Gehazi?' And he said, 'Your servant has not gone anywhere. But he said to him, 'Did I not go with you in spirit when that man returned from his chariot to meet you? Was this an occasion for you to take silver and to take garments, olive groves and vineyards, sheep and oxen, male and female servants? Therefore, Naaman's leprosy will stick to you*

My prayer to the readers of this book is that, if there are still undiscovered impurities in your heart, especially those that destroy the primacy and understanding that God must be First, from the beginning to the end of your story, you may be washed by the Holy Spirit until your spiritual "skin" becomes as clean and smooth as that of a child who listens to and obeys his parents' commands. And may your choices be thought out and decided under the guidance of God's Spirit in you.

Surely there are many things set apart, reserved and promised for you. No matter what it is: whether it's a miracle, healing, financial resources, a relationship or that lawsuit that seeks to destabilize your faith, just rest in God, do what needs to be done and believe until the end. Someone can be used, even an unknown "girl" or anyone who doesn't know you. However, give up what has not been set apart, reserved and kept especially for you, because even if you receive it, it will not come with the blessing and approval that generate durability and multiplication.

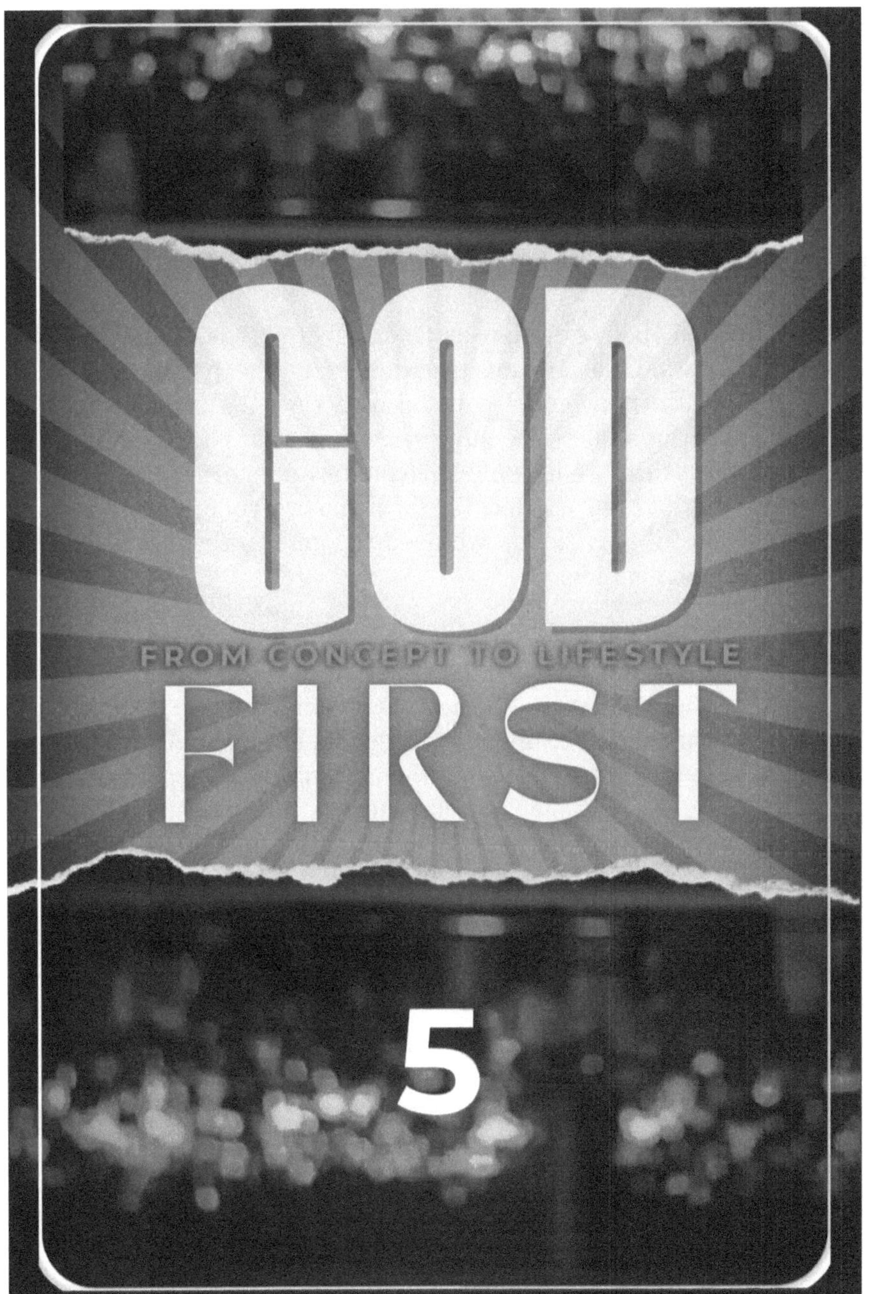

GOD
FROM CONCEPT TO LIFESTYLE
FIRST
5

5 - PARADIGMS AND OTHER TRUTHS

Our daily experiences feed us with what we call paradigms. Having a paradigm is like having a pattern, a model, a norm or a rule; it's a set of forms that shape our perception. That's why it's essential to find out which models and norms have influenced us since birth. If they're good, great! But if they're not, we need to work on them and correct them.

Normally, a person experiences realities that they never expected or imagined. The most unusual and challenging situations throughout life can shape the paradigms that sustain everyone. Thus, in this process of experimentation, which involves both desirable and undesirable situations, the truths we face to survive emerge from the pains and victories that make up our history. Once formed, these models can influence our lives in positive or negative ways, becoming weapons that slow us down or propel us forward.

But here's the question: am I here on Earth just to survive, bound by what I believe to be the truths and limitations that surround me? Or should my intention be to live abundantly, as promised in the Word? The Bible constantly reminds us that *"we are more than conquerors"*, that *"the conquerors through Christ are free from death and the Devil",* that *"the conquerors will march in a triumphal parade and have their names written in the Book of Life forever",* and that *"the conquerors will sit with me at the head of the table... and inherit all this. I will be God to them".* [10]

Every day, I must make a choice: either my humanity stops and focuses on what the devil has to offer, or I decide to live the life that Christ offers me:

"The thief comes only to steal and kill and destroy; I have come that they may have life, and have it to the full." [John 10.10]

True Victory in Christ

We talk a lot about seeking victory, but what should really happen? It is essential to deconstruct the idea of personal victory and emphasize what we have already received: in Christ Jesus, we are more than conquerors. This is the foundation of our faith, anchored in the work of redemption that has already been accomplished. A victory in an earthly lifestyle can never detract from what happened on the cross. The cross is our greatest victory and reward, and any achievement should only be celebrated when our love and surrender to God surpasses our earthly accomplishments.

Believe that you are more than a winner! However, it is essential to examine what is stored inside you.

What is not good must be urgently worked on to achieve complete restoration. Believing in the God who commands and dominates implies recognizing the importance of not ignoring the One who created us and paid a high price for us. It's as if God put an invisible sign on our foreheads that says: "It's paid for, working on my paradigms!"

Once we open ourselves to and transformation and recognize that God is First, we realize that some - or many - of our truths need to be readjusted. In this process, we must place ourselves at the disposal of the Builder, resting and believing that He will complete His work. The reform will be carried out by those who truly understand who we are.

The True Essence of Victory

Thus, true victory does not lie in earthly conquests, but in surrendering to God and accepting the work He does in us. By focusing on redemption and inner transformation, we find a lifestyle that reflects true victory in Christ. This victory - regardless of the circumstances - enables us to live with purpose, joy and a deep connection with the Creator, allowing us to face life's challenges with faith and confidence.

Therefore, as we seek true victory, let us remember that it is not measured by external achievements, but by our willingness to surrender to God and allow Him to work in our lives. This surrender is what transforms us and makes us truly victorious.

But what reform? what restoration? what paradigm shift? In this process I'm in, everything must be confronted, even if it's not entirely comfortable. There is work to be done if I am to succeed, and lots of it! Ken Eldred and George Barna point out that, in many parts of the world, a large part of a person's identity, as well as their deepest truths, is defined by the work they dedicate themselves to. For me, as a Christian, my identity is defined by my faith in God. However, there is a widespread perception among Christians and churches that work in the marketplace has very little intersection with this faith. "The problem with Christianity is not the content of the faith, but the failure of its adherents to integrate the principles of the faith into their lifestyles."[11]

It is important to remember that work is not the result of Adam and Eve's sin; it is part of the original structure since creation and is directly linked to humanity's identity and purpose. My work is not just about bringing home bread; it also involves managing my spirit, soul and body.

Every reform I set out to make, whether in society or on an individual level, requires faith and rest, as well as commitment, work and a lot of patience to finish what has been started. Even so, faith can never be disassociated from the effort that will be required. In the work of rebuilding paradigms, there will be mess, dirt, adjustments and unexpected changes. It may seem that at certain points on the journey I'm parked in different and inhospitable places, when in fact I'm just going through the process of maturing, which is perfectly expected of every son or daughter of God.

Paradigms, therefore, can dictate our personal commitment and surrender, revealing the obvious results of the work in relationships with the people around us. When I read that God gave seeds to the sower, I understand that they were not seeds to be kept and accumulated as personal treasure. The skills and abilities of each human being, as well as the truths we accept, serve as instruments for building God's kingdom in every place we step foot and in the environments we touch.

In my hands, I bear the responsibility for everything that has been entrusted to me individually. If the paradigms generated and assimilated are not correct or are not aligned with the principles of the Word, I can be led to take someone in directions that deviate from the biblical pattern, compromising the purposes for which each person was created. On the other hand, as we have seen, once the truths are aligned, the influence will be positive. Paradigms from the right perspective serve as tools that propel people to unimaginable advances.

Now, pay attention: you are both the storer of the seeds you receive from God and the distributor of that crop to your generation. That's why I say that the spiritual resources for each mission are channeled into people who accept the challenges of their journey. This is how God works when we take steps of faith. Yes, everyone will be rewarded by becoming an instrument of blessing for others. This understanding explains why we want to be more like God: the exercise of giving diminishes the power of evil and breaks the cycle of sin in which the world lives. And this is a work of surrender.

"I have shown you in everything that, working in this way, you must help those in need and remember the words of the Lord Jesus himself: It is more blessed to give than to receive." [Acts 20:35]

Practicing generosity

One of the central objectives of this reconstruction of thought is to cultivate a generous heart. Generosity represents a paradigm shift that I have tried to understand and integrate into my daily life. Each person can develop their own pattern of generosity, but beware: concepts, rules and verses that we learn remain only in the mind if they are not practiced in our routine.

Juliana always intrigued me with her generosity, which seemed excessive to me. After more than two decades of marriage, I questioned her whenever she decided to give away something of greater value or that she had recently acquired. Without realizing it, I was acting like a professional churchgoer. I had to review my concepts, compare them with the principles of the Bible and learn from everything I ministered. Like her, I began to practice generosity more intentionally and repeatedly. For Ju, generosity is a mission; for many, it can be a regular and joyful practice. So I decided to listen to the voice of the Holy Spirit and seek a balance in my generosity, which brought me peace with God.

"The wicked borrow and do not repay, but the righteous give generously..." [Psalms 37.21]

"Happy is the man who lends generously and conducts his business honestly." [Psalms 112.5]

I once dropped my wife off at a doctor's surgery and, as it was going to be a quick visit, I planned to pick her up at a nearby pet store. I went to take care of some other business and came back to find her. As I parked and got out of the car, a nice young man approached me, asking if I would like to buy some Honey Buns to help with his social work. "Not today, my dear!" I replied, heading into the store. But I thought: if I'd been with Ju, she would have stopped to buy the honey buns.

In less than two minutes, we found ourselves in the store and I saw that she had already paid for the snacks for Zeeke, our little Boston Terrier - who, let's face it, looks more like a mixture of a bat and an otter (and let that observation remain between us! lol). Before we left, she said to me: "There's a boy outside selling sweets. Don't you want to bless him? Do you have any change with you? I understood the message and rushed off to do what I should have done, fulfilling my little mission, not before I also heard what the Spirit was saying to me: "I spoke to you to buy from him!"

It sounds simple, but that's how I've been trained in generosity and spiritual listening. Limitations arise because we often don't stop to meditate and discern what we already know and how we can practice it. In addition, we are reminded by the Holy Spirit who dwells in us, who makes us aware of our role as children of God. God's generosity in me is what really matters. Whenever I help someone in need, they thank God, and their act becomes part of their expression of gratitude. Both the recipient is blessed, and the recipient is an open channel for God's love to flow.

What will motivate me to be more grateful and to look like Jesus for everything I receive, regardless of my current situation? Whether rich, middle class or struggling to get anywhere, we are all small channels through which blessings must flow, because there will always be someone with a greater need than ours.

Generosity has no past! When I understood this truth, my entire present and future were transformed. In heaven, my name isn't registered as a person on probation or parole. There is no one watching my every move to take me to prison if I make a mistake at any point. I have received a verdict, my sentence has been paid, and I walk free and without handcuffs. My joy in bearing fruit and sharing in this multiplication comes precisely because something has changed in me; today I have life, joy, abundance and rest in spirit, soul and body.

"To him who gives liberally, more and more will be added; to him who withholds more than is just, it will be to his pure loss. A generous soul will prosper, and he who gives to drink will be fed." [Proverbs 11.24]

Generosity is a daily choice, a reflection of our willingness to serve and love. May we always remember that by giving, we are not only blessing others, but also allowing ourselves to experience the abundance that God has promised.

My friend Joshua!

For a while during my teenage years, my father and his dear friend Joshua ran a fleet of cabs in Brasilia, the capital of Brazil. Although the business wasn't as profitable as planned, that never mattered. We were like a family, and one of my fondest memories of that time is Josué's attitude - always cheerful, generous and fun at my father's side, involved in church work.

But then, unexpectedly and to everyone's surprise, Joshua suffered a stroke and was rushed to hospital. A few years earlier, I had lost my paternal grandfather, and at that moment I didn't want to lose another loved one. Fate has its ways, and our friend passed away in hospital, leaving me deeply shaken. I thought about the children who were my soccer friends; I thought about my father and the pain of losing his faithful companion of so many years. Josué simply left our lives overnight. What I didn't want to forget, however, was their lifestyle and the strong relationship they built with the many families that my father Osmar - now in the nineties - and Joshua looked after with so much love. Nothing was lacking, no one was in need.

The cab fleet with the DKVs and VW Beetles has ended, but the experience and the bonds that existed between them have left me with great memories of what it's like to have a true friend full of generosity. The bonds forged at that time remain, even with the physical distance. They are friends who share struggles and joys, who seek to understand and see each other grow, who support each other when they face difficulties. That time has passed, I've grown up, left the country, matured. But memories like these forge people who are prepared and determined to win. With every new friend I make, I try to draw inspiration from those examples, becoming generous, dedicated and reliable like them. I certainly had a school of life that taught me this zeal, and I try to pass it on to my generation.

...

Many years passed and, already in the São Paulo region, I received a call from Pedrinho, my cousin: *"You may stop looking, I've found a little car for you!"*. After more than 10 years away from Brazil, studying and working, I'd always dreamed that if I came back, I'd buy an old VW and renovate it. I didn't want to have a fleet of cabs like Joshua and my father, but the idea of a VW Beetle appealed to me. That memory took me back to ancient times, to the comings and goings of Brasília, when my parents decided it was time to visit relatives. Our adventure began crammed into the back seat, where the three brothers fought for space, while my father drove us along the bumpy highways that connected our home to the new capital. Brasília was inaugurated in 1960, and our family moved there in 1962, along unpaved roads full of detours. That's why my attraction to the VW has always been strong.

After some negotiations, I made an appointment with Pedrinho in Sorocaba, paid for the car and, with great care and happiness, returned to São Paulo. The white 1970s VW required a lot of work. Over time, I changed the suspension, installed electronic ignition, sealed the holes in the chassis and replaced the old seats. The smell of gasoline still hung in the air, and the choking of the engine, so peculiar to old cars, instigated me even more.

My son Lutti, who was 6 at the time, watched with joy as his dad prepared a special car for him. Many times, when I got home, I ran straight to see what else needed to be restored. I changed the wheels, did some of the bodywork, replaced the carpet and interior, put green film on the windows and installed new steering. The years went by, and my little beetle was almost ready. I was happy, always on the lookout for what else could be done to improve it. I started visiting vintage car fairs, dreaming that, at some point, my car would be there, ready to be judged and awarded.

One day, however, I began to realize in my mind that the Beetle was slipping out of my hands. I couldn't understand or accept why it didn't have such an emotional hold on me. Then a phrase began to echo inside me: *"It's not yours anymore!"*. As a good pastor, I rebuked that thought; something like that couldn't come from above! After all, I had worked hard on the car and made many changes to get it to that condition. The document was in my name; I preached and told everyone how much I loved it and how rightfully I had earned that right. But the phrase kept resounding: *"It's not yours anymore!"*. *"Of course it's not!"*, I defended myself, *'I'm just fixing it up to give to my son!'*. He had fun with me in the renovation, and we drove around the city together. The car had already appreciated in value and many people stopped to admire the restoration.

By then, we no longer lived in São Paulo; our gaze and purposes had shifted to Barueri, where Deus Primeiro was established. And here, a friend enters the story. He came from far away to attend our meetings, usually arriving tired, late or absent on a few occasions, because his car always had mechanical problems. Sometimes the battery didn't work, other times there were problems with the alternator, or the tire went flat. You know where this conversation leads.

One Saturday, he and I were sitting around discussing matters related to the ministry, our covenant, our purposes and the big dreams we've always wanted to achieve. During our conversation, I said, without thinking: *"I'm going to give you the beetle!"*. I was startled; that phrase came out unexpectedly. I didn't think, it wasn't in context, I just said it! He smiled, not understanding what was happening. At that moment, I thought: *"What a crazy word! I'm not well! I'm being carried away by my emotions! That's not sensible, after all, I've invested a lot more than I paid for this car!"*. But the phrase echoed again: *"It's not yours anymore!"*, and I finally understood what the Holy Spirit was communicating to me.

Then something incredible happened: I felt an undeniable and definitive peace. I didn't need to understand it, because I couldn't even if I tried. Now at peace and fulfilled, I realized that the story was coming to an end - only to begin a new and even better one! My emotions stopped fighting against something that was a fait accompli in a place deeper than my soul. I got home and slept well! Relieved, happy and, once again, fulfilled! We arranged a day for the pastor to pick up the car, and I talked to Ju and my son. I felt that when I put my emotions aside to fulfill something I had heard from God, my son didn't mind either. Of course, if we can, someday we'll restore a little car just for us.

Without realizing it, I was establishing a legality that transferred the same blessing and condition to my home. In all honesty, I felt like I was acquiring, preparing and handing over something that had been placed in my hands only to multiply and give back to God's kingdom. This time, it would be for someone who needed it much more than I did. My friend, soon after, managed to sell the beetle and his car, acquiring a much better automobile. It was also a moment of God for him and his wife, and they soon had a son.

I could see how our heavenly Father works. He gives us the joy of achieving what we imagine, he gives us the health to manage the harvest process, and he expects us to do the right thing at harvest time, just when he tells us to sow the seeds. It could be a little car, a job, a lot or a little money, investments; none of it is really ours. God only waits for a heart decision to honor and multiply.

We will always have opportunities and gifts from God that help us understand and live more about giving, letting go, investing, multiplying and sowing. Jesus Christ gave us the greatest example by teaching us to look after and care for others, even outside his world. He left the kingdom of God, as Son and heir, to come and live like us. So, we can see that everything happens under a careful plan from God, with details that allow us to act and become instruments of blessing.

In my beetle story, there is no pride involved, except that which was broken by thinking I could control the situation, believing that *"it was mine!"*. My joy in recognizing that I can share what I consider mine is much greater when I place it in the Father's hands. My truths can change whenever they are confronted or presented in the light of the Word. God will cause the things around us to be adjusted for the favor and blessings that have already been reserved, stored, prepared and directed for an end that He knows best.

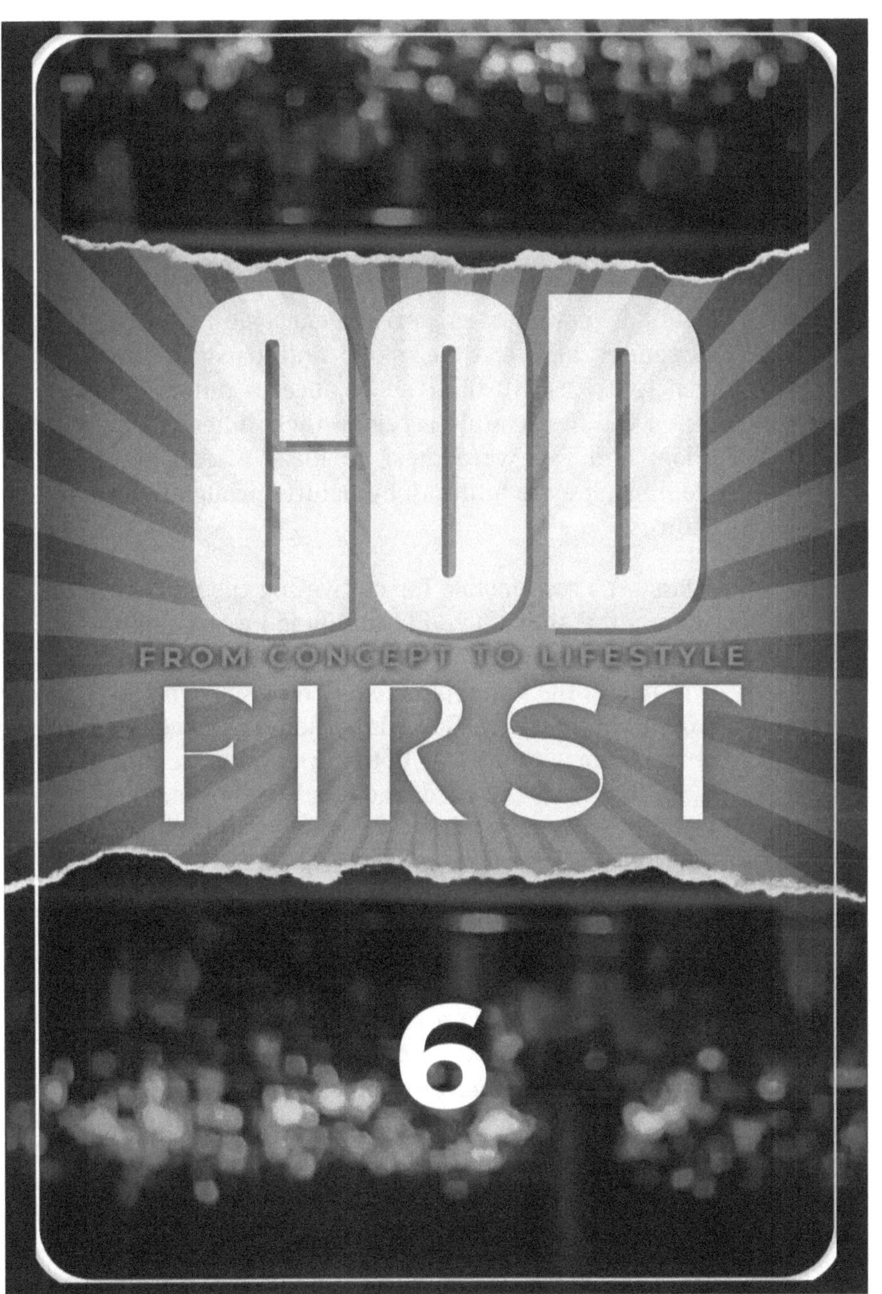

GOD
FROM CONCEPT TO LIFESTYLE
FIRST
6

6 – WHOSE IDEA WAS IT?

From the beginning of the Bible, we learn that giving is not just an act of generosity; it is a surrender of life, time, skills and trust in the principles that sustain the balance of humanity. When the first couple received their inheritance, Adam and Eve were there to blaze a trail that would shape the future of humanity through their choices.

Adam was responsible for cultivating the garden, naming the animals and faithfully following God's instructions. Eve, created from Adam's rib, symbolizes the union planned by God for man and woman in marriage. God's intention was never to tempt them with the fruit of that tree, but to reminf them that He is the Lord, and it is He who sets the standards we must follow. Mike Hayes, in his book "When God is First", reminds us that:

> "The tree of Knowledge of Good and Evil was supposed to be a constant reminder that, even with power anda authority, they were still commanded by another being. The first ste towards the fall was forgetting its foundation."

Unfortunately, the human tendency is to make decisions based on the desires of the soul, rather than listening to the voice of the spirit, often without reflecting on the consequences and the principles we have received. Despite the perfect structure and care that God had prepared, we saw the negligence of Adam and Eve, who allowed themselves to be deceived, ignoring the advice they had received. The concepts and the whole structure were in place, but the lifestyle depended on the couple. If they, who didn't have a thousandth of the distractions and influences we face today, were deceived by the enemy's talk, it makes us reflect on the importance of trusting and depending on what we have already been taught.

We understand that structure generates behavior. On the other hand, a lack of structure can generate unbalanced behavior. Cain and Abel grew up under the influence of their parents' behavior. Cain, for his part, accepted selfish behavior and had to bear the consequences of his mistakes. Like Adam and Eve, Cain was guided by the desires and emotions of the soul, while Abel offered his offering with a grateful and generous heart, and his offering was blessed by God. Abel chose not to be carried away by uncertainties and doubts, because his spirit was open to listening and allowing the best to be generated in him. Although Abel lost his life, he didn't stop obeying and did everything in his power.

God is the inventor of generosity and surrender. It was He who gave His Son, Jesus, to pay the price and redeem us from the fatal error that originated in Eden.

Generosity is a practice that transcends the simple act of giving; it is an attitude of the heart. When we open ourselves to this truth, we transform not only our lives, but also the lives of those around us. Every act of generosity is a seed planted that can bear abundant fruit.

So how are you cultivating your generosity? Are you willing to give up what you consider yours to bless others? Remember that in doing so, we are not only following Christ's example, but also becoming instruments of His grace and love in this world.

Giving is a daily choice, a reflection of our willingness to serve and love. May we always remember that by giving, we are not only blessing others, but also allowing ourselves to experience the abundance that God has

Here you plant, here you reap

Robert Morris clarifies this matter crystal clear and conclusively: *"If God is the subject and we are the object, then the verb 'to give' is what completes the sentence. Most people can argue and say 'no'! But the verb in the Bible is 'love', because God is love!"*. We read in John 3:16 that God loved so much that he gave. If He only loved, we wouldn't be here discussing the subject. So, by giving, he rewards us so that we can reward others around us. Our generosity of time will, and financial resources contributes to the growth of the kingdom. We give ourselves physically, perhaps to the point of exhaustion, but all the giving involved in fulfilling our role in establishing the kingdom on earth is a demonstration that we are integrally part of the Master's work.

"And this I say, he who sows sparingly shall reap sparingly; and he who sows bountifully shall reap bountifully. Let everyone give as he has purposed in his heart, not grudgingly or of necessity; for God loves a cheerful giver. God is able to make you abound in every grace, so that always having ample sufficiency in all things, you may abound in every good work, as it is written: he distributed, he gave to the poor, his righteousness endures forever. Now he who gives seed to the sower and bread for food will also supply and increase your sowing and multiply the fruits of your righteousness, enriching you in everything for all generosity, which causes thanks to be rendered to God through us." [2Corinthians 9:6-11]

From a non believer's point of view, it's hard to believe that God cares about meeting humanity's needs. After all, if we stop to focus our attention on some countries, it seems that God doesn't even exist - that's how many people think! However, we forget to reflect on the most conservative aspect: all of creation is His work.

> *"The earth is the Lord's, and all that is in it, the world and those who live in it; for it is he who has established it above the seas and made it firm above the waters.... He who has clean hands and a pure heart, who does not turn to idols or swear by false gods. He will receive blessings from the Lord, and God his Savior will do him justice..."* [Psalms 24.1,2,4,5]

That makes it easier to understand, because that's how every father likes it: to take care of his children, his generation, his successors and representatives; those who will carry his name forward. Another point is that any reward we may receive - even if we don't deserve it - comes about because if our mission to give and be generous is fulfilled, He receives it with joy. This irrationality, which the world sees as madness - that we are loved more for giving than for receiving - defies all the economics textbooks in any university in the world. It would be very difficult to expect Einstein to come up with a human formula that could explain this truth.

For a long time, I justified my insecurity by saying: *"We can give more when we are more secure and financially stable!"*. The statement is coherent, and each person must assess their limitations. But this is not the same as using our limitations as a crutch of excuses, preventing us from serving others.

Wasn't that how the disciples complained about the perfumed oil the woman used to wash Jesus' feet? *"We could have sold this alabaster jar and given the money to the poor!"*. How false! They were criticizing for the sake of criticizing, judging for the sake of judging. But that's what we do when we close our eyes and sit comfortably on our sofas!

Take advantage of these examples, use them as tools, use them to develop daily habits and to structure your earnings correctly. Our behavior will always reflect the structure we rely on.

I believe that you too will "convert" to what God has already established from the beginning. He wants the best for everyone, because he knows that we have been deceived and succumbed to the system that is devouring us. See how this generation walks like distracted sheep, constantly being deceived and accepting what is easiest.

Generosity is a daily choice, a reflection of our willingness to serve and love. May we always remember that by giving, we are not only blessing others, but also allowing ourselves to experience the abundance that God has promised.

...

The concept of putting God first in our lives has been sown since creation, from the moment we accepted Christ as Lord. It was on that day that we received the most precious gift there is: the certainty that all our sins have been forgiven! The mere thought of *"Then I'll give!"* is proof that there is a seed of generosity planted inside you, ready to sprout at any moment. However you look at it, God has already deposited generosity in us even before the foundation of the world.

> *"For God so loved the world that he gave his one and only Son, that whoever believes in him shall not perish but have eternal life."* [John 3.16]

One of the reasons why millions of people don't understand this message is that they believe the focus is on them. However, the fundamental subject of the Scriptures is God, and we are only the object of the Bible, rescued and saved from the doom of hell, even if we don't deserve it.

From Generation to Generation

Think of the children born into the same family. I have three daughters and a son. Four people, each with their own way and personality, seeking their own faith and lifestyle. My siblings and I also grew up hearing the truths of the principles of God's Word. However, all of us, including my children, went through times when we wanted to rule the universe in our own way. It took time to discover that we are not the center of the galaxy. We have learned to move from fear mode to faith mode! Each in their own way, but all grounded in the same principles and truths of the Word.

At the age of 19, I was given the opportunity to take an Evangelism and Leadership course in San Diego, California, sponsored by Evangelist Morris Cerullo. Fifty other Brazilians and I had the privilege of studying with more than six hundred people from many nations, living with customs and personalities very different from our own. It was a unique culture experience, but one that left its mark on my heart: the desire to serve God like never before in my life.

After spending nine months outside Brazil, I received an invitation to train people together with the leaders of the Student Crusade in Brasilia. I dedicated myself for a whole year, visiting and training teams in dozens of churches in the Federal District. During this training, we prepared a team for a major evangelistic campaign, focused on distributing thousands of leaflets on the "4 Spiritual Laws", with the aim of reaching 500,000 people in one week. Today, decades later, I am immensely grateful to God for those months and for the blessings that came in the following years. Little did I know that I was being prepared for higher flights. It reminds me of how Jesus was also tested and learned:

"Although he was a Son, he learned obedience through his suffering. By this he was enabled to be the perfect High Priest and became the source of eternal salvation for all who obey him." [Hebrews 5.8-9]

The value of self-giving is a theme that permeates the Christian life. It is fundamental to understand that, when we give, we are not just fulfilling a duty but participating in a divine plan that connects us to each other and brings us closer to God.

God calls us to live this truth, and with every act of generosity, we are not only blessing others, but also allowing ourselves to experience the abundance that He has promised. May we always remember that by giving, we are contributing to the growth of His kingdom and becoming instruments of His grace and love in this world.

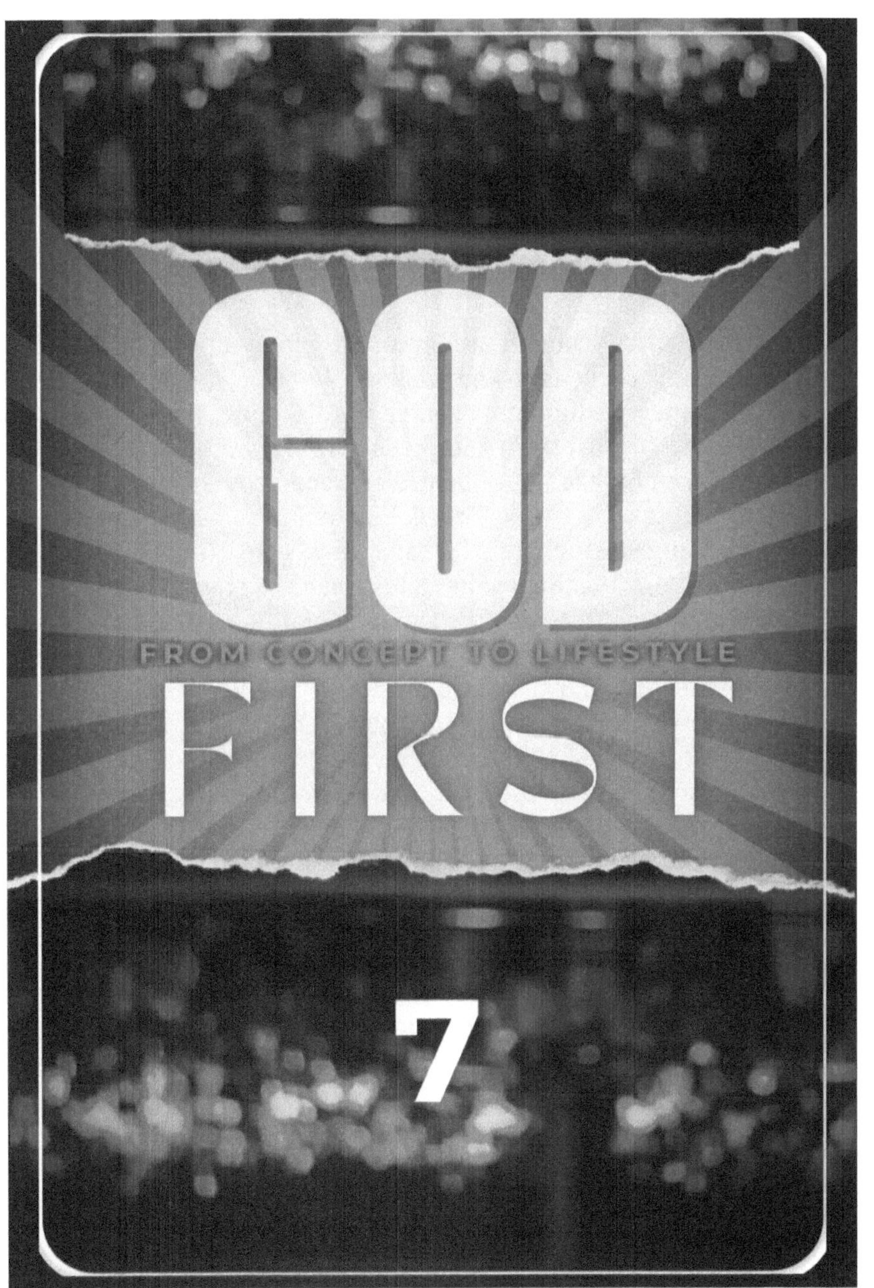

GOD
FROM CONCEPT TO LIFESTYLE
FIRST
7

7 - TITHING, MUCH MORE THAN A BOGEYMAN!

When we convert to Christ, we often come with many challenges and doubts. When it comes to money, we think that people are dishonest, that it's hard to trust them and that's why we want to take care of what's ours before someone comes along and takes it away. This is how many come to the evangelical church. Juliana, my wife, uses an analogy that helped her a lot when she started out in the church with the same mentality. She heard the following comparison: "Think that every time you give your tithe or offering, it's as if you were a straw through which God blows. You don't know exactly what happens on the other end; you don't know if the person will make good use of it, but your part is to be the straw. The word must pass through you to create the effect it can generate."

Tithing is a subject that always generates a lot of discussion and, unfortunately, is often trivialized in the history of the Church, even though the Bible is full of examples of the importance of obeying God's law of sowing and reaping.   This truth is unquestionable.

Many people dwell on the details and how to demonstrate a generous and open heart for the things of the kingdom. However, millions of people around the world already enjoy the blessed grace of being able to give back to God what they have received as the fruit of their labor. This individual choice generates inner security and richness of life in all aspects, including financial.

Tithing: God's project for generations

Giving has always been God's project. In the early church, as we read in Acts, there was multiplication from the preaching of the disciples. With each new disciple who accepted the Gospel message, a new lifestyle was grafted in. Each one came forward for multiplication with everything they had, giving generously of their time, talent and possessions. Some gave everything they had, others part of their sales and others financed the work and travel of those who were willing to do a more intense service of sharing.

Today, there are millions of converts on every continent because of that initial church work, and many of them also don't hesitate to give God what is his. However, with great intensity, we see those who seek to minimize the truth of the Word and its principles. For them, tithing seems to be a scheme set up to take some money from the person to leverage illicit enrichment.

Tithing: an immutable Biblical truth

History shows us that corruption knows no bounds, even when it comes to religion. However, we cannot close our eyes to this reality. The actions of acknowledging and thanking God for the result of earnings, the fruit of work and sweat, have persisted among the faithful since the beginning of time.

Even in the face of individual questioning and human concepts that seek to inhibit the actions of people of faith within the house of God, the fundamental basis of the teaching of tithes and offerings has been maintained throughout the centuries, because the Bible has not changed. So what has changed? The mere mention of tithing has become the terror of the unbeliever and, if there is a lack of understanding, a bogeyman for the believer himself.

Over the last 60 years or so, much has changed in the diabolical attempt to promote biblical deconstruction. Many are rising to question and challenge the very foundations of the Gospel that have sustained us until now. Our children and this whole generation have been exposed very quickly to all kinds of information through smartphones, the internet, educational institutions and, of course, the humanist and opportunistic media.

As a result, society has received a flood of teachings meticulously inserted into educational systems, leveraged by socialism.

The strategy, for us, has been clearly exposed and it turns against the family and fundamental traditional bases. In the development and expansion of this global society and culture of which we are a part, two systems of thought have emerged as the most pronounced and influential.

Conflict between two systems

First, there is the Judeo-Christian biblical and cultural system, where God established the initial rules. These guidelines are firmly rooted in Scripture and, even after the fall of man, the teaching has been passed down from father to son, through generations to the present day.

The emergence of humanist thought

In contrast, we have the second system, which we can call humanist, originating from Greek thought. This arose with the aim of producing rational knowledge about nature. Unlike Judeo-Christian thought, humanists were never nurtured in the knowledge of the God of creation and believed in many gods.

These systems clash and, why not say it, clash constantly, which is why we will never find unanimity between Thales of Miletus, Heraclitus of

Ephesus and Pythagoras and what the biblical prophets heard and wrote to us about God. The basis of Genesis 1 does not coincide with what Zeus, Poseidon or Aphrodite say, for example. Obviously, they didn't understand sin or how to erase it from their lives, which is why the Greeks thought that the gospel of Christ was foolish. To understand them better, look at what modern society thinks about the gospel of Christ:

"So, when we preach that Christ was crucified, the Jews are offended, and the Gentiles say it is foolishness." [1 Corinthians 1:23-NVT]

However, by allowing itself to be carried away by excess and extremism, the godless society moved away from the foundations of the first system, concentrating its forces on pure human development. It thus disregarded the primacy of God in the most fundamental aspects of life. Divine thought was gradually replaced by great philosophers and little gods, who distorted the essential truths established by the Creator.

Nothing new under the sun!

The Greek humanist system of thought is nothing new. Its revolutionary ideas have been spreading across the globe since long before Christ came to Earth. The Epicureans believed that man evolved from the earth itself, from the ground he walked on, and consequently their philosophy was profoundly materialistic.

The spread of the teachings

Over the centuries, the teachings of these two systems spread throughout the world. If you lived in the early 1960s, as I did, you certainly experienced the exploitation of ideas and transformations that the prince of this world has accelerated more than ever. This strategy of the devil is not new; it began in Eden, but is now manifesting itself at this alarming speed, taking advantage of the lack of modesty and spiritual degradation that is very evident on the continents we tread. Looking at what is happening, we can say that we are living in days that rival those of Sodom and Gomorrah.

The evil strategy at work

For centuries, as we have seen, this evil strategy has been at work in the minds of men and women, in educational institutions and within homes, destroying the value of the family.

It infiltrates research and demonizes the creationist system, with the collaboration of governments that bow to men of low character.

These governments establish laws that lead people with a lower capacity for discernment to the spiritual and, consequently, intellectual precipice.

Just look at the growing and very influential despair of the progressive Woke culture. A political term of African American origin, which derives from the English vernacular *"stay woke"*, and whose main struggle is linked to issues of social and racial justice, but in an invidious way. We have observed that even though it has been accepted by society in many countries and organizations from the most diverse sectors, little by little, many companies that initially showed support are beginning to stop extending support, due to the weakness of their ideas and the extremism of their thinking. It is easy for us Christians to discern the anti-Christian tendency.

The aim of this society has been very clear: to subtly make people begin to question the veracity of God's Word, casting unfounded doubts in the minds of young people, the biggest victims of this neglect.

The devaluation of Creation

Over time, biblical aspects of essential importance have been subtly undermined. Creation is challenged and increasingly minimized in educational systems, while the theory of evolution - just a **t-h-e-o-r-y** - is masterfully promoted by humanist marketers, even without compelling evidence. These architects of evolutionism are the same progressives who stand up against the solid parameters of the Bible.

So, the battle between these two systems of thought continues, but it is up to us, as conscientious individuals, to discern and resist the influences that seek to distort the truth. The fight for the integrity of God's Word and the valorization of divine principles is more relevant than ever.

Despite all the challenges, the truth about tithing remains unchanged, because it has purpose. It is up to each of us, as faithful followers of Christ, to understand and practice this biblical truth, not letting tithing become a bogeyman, but rather an expression of our love and gratitude to God.

The quest for relativization

Incredible as it may seem, the desire to re-signify or re-edit the Bible has even been considered by so-called evangelical leaders. Perhaps, to relativize, these leaders prefer to live without transformation. Many of these leaders, apparently influenced by the media or out of sheer spiritual blindness, discuss how much 'evolution' can be boxed into the Bible to satisfy their followers. Things like this prove that the will of man always seeks to mold itself to what is easiest and least confronting, thus opening doors to critics of the Word. Nominal believers also fall into this trap - and not necessarily neophytes - who, because they don't have a depth of understanding, are almost always deceived and mix the essence of the Word with a mixture of their own poison.

The importance of worship

It is commendable and we need to rejoice in the millions of believers who seek God around the world, but there will always be a condition:

> *"The Spirit of God dwells in you. And if anyone does not have the Spirit of Christ, he is not his."*
> [Romans 8.9]

At the same time, churches justify themselves by having large numbers of members, without worrying about what they present to the society in which they live. We can understand why there is so much hatred towards believers who support this Gospel. But which is more important? The financial result or being prostrate in worship, filled with the Holy Spirit? Yes, nothing we see today comes as a surprise. The confrontation between the humanist system and Judeo-Christian thought is ancient, and it is up to us, as faithful followers of Christ, to hold firm to the condition of faith, resisting the temptations to relativize the Word of God. The answer lies in prostrating ourselves in adoration of the Creator, putting aside worldly concerns and giving ourselves completely to Him.

All truth is parallel

The late American evangelist Morris Cerullo said that all truth is parallel. If evil strategies have risen and taken over the most diverse fronts of society, so too has the Gospel been spread throughout the world, with the same authority and efficiency as always. If the enemy side has a strategy, the strategies that God gives will be better and more effective.

When Paul proclaimed the Gospel to the Greeks of the time, and knowing that they would not understand the message of one God, the same message that was preached to the Jews, he maintained the established principles and foundations, but changed the mental path of persuasion:

"To the lawless, as though I myself were lawless, not being without law toward God, but under the law of Christ, to win those who live outside the law. I made myself weak toward the weak in order to win the weak. I have made myself all things to all people in order to save some by all means. I do everything for the sake of the gospel, so that I may cooperate with it." [1 Cor 9.21-23]

Paul addressed the Greeks with the Gospel in a spectacular manner, and even while speaking of God, he used what was familiar to them. He spoke of their unknown god, which became a strategic element in his preaching. Paul took advantage of this approach to convert them and bring about life changes. He used common facts, such as blood—the blood we inherit from Adam—discussed sin and the need for salvation, and influenced those with an evolutionary mindset, challenging Greek thought and form by utilizing a Christian foundation.

"The natural man does not accept the things of the Spirit of God, for they are foolishness to him; nor can he know them, because they are spiritually discerned." [1 Corinthians 2:14]

Repentance as key

When we study examples of life transformation through the preaching of the Word, especially concerning finances, generosity, tithes, and offerings, we can distill the message into one word: repentance. Repentance for having thought and lived according to our own ideas and truths, beyond what we learned from others, when we should initially pay attention to the Word.

Responding to the Challenge

In recent generations, both in Brazil and in countries with a strong evangelical presence, we observe a concerning phenomenon. As social and political systems clash and churches fail to adequately fulfill their roles, many people have been exposed to superficial and shallow knowledge tailored to their personal feelings and desires. Furthermore, when biblical teaching occurs, it often comes with interpretations and human opinions that cannot be fully substantiated by Scripture.

As part of the solution rather than the problem, we need to act wisely in favor of the Gospel, perhaps adopting strategies like those of the Apostle Paul. Likewise, while society debates issues like abortion, we can raise discussions about the value and meaning of life. Considering rising immorality and pornography, we can strengthen teachings on moral standards by introducing principles that transform the mindset of those around us.

While the world succumbs to homosexuality and promiscuity—leading to consequences like illegitimacy—the Church must courageously proclaim with fervor the values and importance of family. Simultaneously, we should demonstrate love and compassion for those involved in these situations so that they may become children of God.

It is fundamental for the Church to assume its role as a spiritual and moral guide in society, offering solid and transformative biblical teaching. At the same time, we must act with wisdom, love, and compassion so that we can be instruments of change and reconciliation in an increasingly challenging world.

> *"But if you seek God and plead with the Almighty, if you are pure and upright, even now he will rouse himself for you and restore your rightful place."* [Job 8:5-6]

Despite observing governments that succumb to their own laws, we can still believe that we will have Christian professionals, such as lawyers, doctors, academics, and politicians, who are not ashamed to ensure that law and peace prevail. When we perceive that human opinion seeks to dominate social or ideological discourse, we must use God's Word as a guide and foundation. Finally, when the theory of evolution presents its lies, it must be demolished by the love of creation.

This is the lifestyle I'm talking! It is the result of putting God first, always. By doing so, we become salt and light in the world, positively influencing society and defending the values of the Kingdom of God.

It is essential for us to assume our responsibilities in all spheres of society, using our faith as a basis for all actions and decisions. Only then can we be agents of transformation and witness the power of the Gospel amid an increasingly challenging world.

Clear advice!

One of the clearest and most direct verses about our responsibility to sponsor the Gospel of Christ and donate without humanistic impediments or interference is, surprisingly, in the New Testament. The Apostle Paul addressed the need of the church in Jerusalem and emphasized how it needed to prepare to advance and fulfill its purpose.

Paul, in his letters, exhorted Christians to be generous and contribute to the support of those in need, especially in times of difficulty. He highlighted the importance of unity among Christians, both Jews and Gentiles, and the need to support one another in love and responsibility. This call to action reflects the essence of the Gospel, which invites us to act with compassion and solidarity, involving all people around us. Each one fulfilling and filling his scope of influence with grace and effectiveness.

So, as we reflect on the role of the church and Christians in society, we must remember the importance of supporting the Gospel selflessly, allowing Christ's message to spread and transform lives:

"Now about the collection for God's people: Do what I told the Galatian churches to do. On the first day of every week, each one of you should set aside a sum of money in keeping with your income, saving it up, so that when I come no

Paul's context

There was a context behind Paul's words. It was not a standard he had decided on just for his support team; it was the custom of the early church. Nor was it a one-time opportunity. The apostle simply reminded the Corinthians of what was already common in the churches of Galatia, confirming an established teaching for future generations. The money raised by the churches was not only for the needs of the apostles. The resources generated were used by ministerial agents in each region, supporting widows and orphans, and serving all who needed it. Thus, they established the foundations of a church that grew and strengthened through each person who delivered their finances, witnessing multiplication before their eyes. "Do not wait until I arrive." This expression makes me reflect on the culture that developed in our church.

With the use of the internet, many of our members are serious before God with their tithes and offerings, not even waiting for Sunday celebrations with their families. Bank transfers are frequently used, and many joyfully fulfill their mission, as they have understood that the first part belongs to the Lord and should not remain in our accounts if we can deliver it in advance.

Remember, we sacrifice the first—which is the Lord's—so that the remainder may be blessed and multiplied, both by our work and, most importantly, by the favor of the Lord upon those who fear Him. Today, just as it was the habit of Christ's disciples, we increasingly concern ourselves with how workers should be compensated for their labor so that they can live dignified lives with their families.

Challenges in sending missionaries

Some experiences from the not-so-distant past in many churches still require care and correction. The practice of "sending" someone to the mission field, both domestically and internationally, often causes more embarrassment than joy, and the results can be disastrous if there is no coherence in leadership. Churches that send their missionaries without studying and evaluating what they may encounter and what their greatest challenges will be can reap undesirable fruits.

As a result, we witness couples who cannot physically or emotionally withstand the calling and return ashamed because their foundation did not prepare them adequately. At some point, these workers find themselves without resources and structure, giving up in the face of the reality they encounter, often with wives and children exposed to despair. One can never know what kind of opposition there will be, but it is essential to take greater care in preparation and suitability.

The struggle of the preacher and the use of resources

The struggle of those who preach the Gospel is greater than one might imagine. The calling may exist, and a person may dedicate themselves wholeheartedly, but difficulties and lack of support can lead even the most courageous preacher to question whether they should continue in their mission. Yes, for Christ we give our lives, and nothing will stop us from moving forward. However, if the church truly focuses on the salvation of people, it is necessary to constantly evaluate how its resources should be used in favor of the Gospel and those involved in the Lord's work.

Your money being multiplied

The result of tithes and offerings should serve to advance the Kingdom of God. Every finance from a Christian organization, whatever it may be, needs to focus its actions primarily on reaching new members. At the same time, but wisely, it should structure places of worship and establish a dignified space for fellowship without ever forgetting those less privileged around us—without making them so dependent on help that they do not seek their own sustenance. It is important to understand that there is no requirement to have gigantic—and idle—buildings to worship God. You and I can worship the Lord under trees, by riversides, or in huts in the middle of the desert. God knows well what goes on in the hearts of His children who worship Him in spirit and truth.

The example of Haggai – A call to action!

Observe how Haggai dealt with the situation of worshiping the Lord. The construction of the altar and temple of the Lord was abandoned. The people had been freed from exile in Babylon and, upon arriving in Judea, found a temple in ruins. Haggai, sent by God, correctly discerned and identified a connection between the community's failure in their areas of work and their neglect of the Lord's temple. His first sermon out of four delivered in this small book from the Old Testament challenged the people to stop prioritizing their personal comfort and to concentrate their efforts on restoring worship to God and rebuilding the temple if they expected to have any success.

We are not here to build our little kingdoms, much less to seek personal success! The obligation of a Christian is to discover, in God and in His Word, the best way to cooperate. Haggai called the people of Jerusalem to true worship, trust in the Word of God, personal holiness, and obedience to the leadership chosen by the Lord. The lifestyle that the people led was not consistent with what would lead them to success. The message is clear: we must commit ourselves to God's work, prioritizing worship and generosity so that we can see the Kingdom of God advance in our lives and communities.

From the right perspective!

When discussing tithes and offerings, even if some argue that this time has passed, it is essential to understand the joy that comes from giving and how it is part of our human nature. We were created for this, and we must honor the Creator by thanking Him for the strength and sustenance we receive from heaven as we live.

A life without God's sustenance and presence will inevitably show us that all our work and effort have been in vain. But a life under God's sustenance and in His presence will bring to light the fruit of everything we have sown!

- Is it hard? It could be worse!
- Is there surplus? It shouldn't be; where do you plan to invest?
- What more do I need to do to see God's work grow?
- Who does more than I do and needs help?

These are fair questions that arise when we seek to return to God what does not belong to us. You might say:*"But if I don't wake up early to work... if I hadn't done every thing I did to finish my degree, it would have been for nothing; God wouldn't do anything."*

Acknowledgment of the First

Yes, your most important moments on the journey to success required effort and hours of hard work. However, true pleasure comes when we discover who is First in everything.

From this point on, the discourse can change: *"If it weren't for God, I wouldn't wake up early, and I wouldn't be able to work; if it weren't for God, I couldn't have done everything I've done..."*

See how the Holy Spirit manifests itself. The prophet Haggai was called to reprimand the people for their lack of interest in worshiping God, calling them to repentance and spiritual renewal. Likewise, the ability to gather and multiply any amount in my hands is not my merit; I am merely a steward of the finances and goods entrusted to me, even if acquired through my own effort, intelligence, and work.

Does having more necessarily mean better? Yes, but only when there is recognition of who is First in my life. Otherwise, I may be consumed by personal pleasures and desires, living without direction or eternal purposes.

God rejoices when we use what He has given us. Remember: when He gave us life and created us, we were born with a generous heart.

The inner struggle with finances

At this point in our conversation, I still do not know how you handle your finances, but it is common for the natural human feeling to be one of retaining more than distributing. To overcome this inner inclination, I face a constant battle to not conform to this world and to not yield to the desires of my soul. By seeking to live under this perspective, I can more easily perceive the misguided way many Christians have managed their finances. It becomes evident that, often without realizing it, people believe they are more competent and skilled in their financial actions than the very God they claim to follow.

The danger of self-sufficiency

The danger of this behavior is that, by challenging their own abilities, they open themselves up to fall indiscriminately into the dungeon of individual loss. Unfortunately, this has been the disastrous lifestyle of many believers who "attend" weekly services. It is important to highlight that attending is different from participating in worship. A simple analysis of this context reveals that human ideas of prosperity and wealth have never been so inferior compared to those we find in the Word of God.

The importance of community

This underscores the importance of the church in each person's life, where everyone is constantly taught and corrected to fulfill their part. Many who persist in seeking the best from God in their journey discover that everything they have does not belong to them; yet they are tremendously blessed and grateful. As we draw closer to the truth, we realize the privilege of existing to enjoy the opportunities to possess goods, multiply what we have, and acquire things through our work and abilities. This happens because He gives us life and allows us all of this, preventing us from stealing glory that we do not deserve.

Awareness and its effects

Without this awareness, life becomes burdensome, doubts arise, distrust increases, and difficulty grows when I reach into my pocket to give "my" money to the church. The reasoning we apply to the church can be the same as what we use for ourselves: "How will I sustain myself if God does not give me the strength for this work?"

Friend, God has done His part, and surely, we can and need to do ours. It is essential to remember that our giving of time and finances has never been established as an obligation but initially as an act of worship and gratitude. Once we are aware that everything, we have is a gift from God, our perspective changes completely. We begin to see giving as an opportunity to honor Him who sustains and blesses us.

May we, together, cultivate this mindset of generosity and gratitude, recognizing that in giving, we are contributing to God's work and aligning ourselves with His purposes.

The concept is not mine!

When the subject is the tithe given in churches, sincere questions, jokes, concepts, and even defamations arise. One of the first doubts that emerges in disbelief is: who brought this idea? We have discussed many concepts and examples about the act of giving and how we can be grateful for everything we receive. What we can affirm is that the concept of tithing was not developed by an advertising agency that knew how to generate desire or fear of scarcity in people's minds. It was not invented by a pastor with a convincing oratory who knows exactly how to touch people's hearts so that they let go of everything "for God." No, the author of this concept is the Lord Himself, Jehovah Jireh – the Provider God – who taught us about the principle of giving. The name of this book says it all: God First!

The meaning of tithing

The word "tithe" means a tenth, or ten percent. So why did God say, "I want you to bring me the first ten percent to my house?" I believe He did this for our own good, not the other way around. This instruction aims to remove selfishness and greed from our hearts, inserting faith in that same space within me and every person who inhabits the Earth. In other words, whenever we give our tithe or any amount to the Lord, it requires faith and trust!

When we study the guidelines God gave to the people of Israel for their success as a nation, He says, "When your sheep have offspring, bring me the first." He did not say, "Wait until your sheep have ten offspring and bring me one of them" or "the one you don't like very much." It does not require faith to give to God what we choose to give. He says, "Bring me the first," even when there are no other nine—and here the concept of firstfruits also comes into play. As we have already understood, God always asks us to sacrifice the first so that He Himself may bless and multiply all the rest.

The principle of putting God First

Here, once again, we see the principle of putting God first being established in our hearts. There is no way to separate this giving, as it involves our entire life:

> *"For where your treasure is, there your heart will be also."* [Matthew 6:21]

This is the greatest evidence of this faith operation. You may say, "But this was a custom of the Old Testament. We are in the dispensation of grace, and I do not have this obligation. It is an ancient principle!" It is necessary to understand that there are principles of God that span both the Old and New Testaments. Even in Malachi 3:10, when it says, *"Bring all the tithes...",* we read in the verses that precede it that God affirms, *"For I the Lord do not change..."* [Malachi 3:6]. The aspects of God's character are eternal and never change. For example, God cannot lie. The reason He cannot lie is that He is the truth! He is not like you and me, who desire—or struggle—to tell the truth. God is the purest expression of truth and therefore cannot lie.

The immutability of the principle

What does this mean? It means that God's principles are eternal and not subject to change according to dispensations. Tithing is not just a religious practice; it reflects a relationship of trust and gratitude to God. When we understand this, our perspective on the act of giving is transformed.

Therefore, when we consider tithing, we should not see it as an obligation but as an opportunity to honor God and recognize that everything we have comes from Him. This shift in mindset not only frees us from fear and scarcity but places us in a position of abundance and blessings, allowing us to live without the fear of dependence on money. We must embrace the concept of tithing as a divine principle that guides us on our faith journey, enabling us to experience the true joy of giving and trusting in the Provider who never fails.

Principles that transform lives

There are principles that, if we observe them, will be a blessing for our entire lives. Jesus taught us: *"You shall not commit adultery!"* Where had He heard or read this? Certainly, in the writings of the Old Testament. But being Jesus, He elevated the responsibility and completed it:

> *"But I tell you that anyone who looks at a woman lustfully has already committed adultery with her in his heart."* [Matthew 5:27-28]

Jesus, full of grace and truth, raised the standard even higher. He wanted you and me to understand that everything relates to the heart! Loving the Lord with all your heart is fundamental. Serving in the church, playing or singing, and even bringing your tithes and offerings—all of this must come from the heart. But why? Because your heart is deceitful and needs to be constantly confronted and corrected.

Similarly, we hear: *"You shall not murder!"*—which means: you shall not kill—but where was that? In the law. And Jesus continued:

> *"You shall love your neighbor as yourself."* [Matthew 19:18-19]

Once again, we see that the work the Holy Spirit expects to accomplish in the hearts of God's children is a solid foundation. Tithing follows the same path, as it is a principle that God used years before the law, and Jesus Himself confirms it in His words. Therefore, we can affirm that it is a principle that permeates Scripture, both in the Old and New Testaments.

> *"Woe to you, teachers of the law and Pharisees, you hypocrites! You give a tenth of your spices—mint, dill, and cumin. But you have neglected the more important matters of the law—justice, mercy, and faithfulness. You should have practiced the latter, without neglecting the former."* [Matthew 23:23]

A Reminder from the past

Let's go back a few years in time. It took me many years to understand, at its core, how managing my money related to my lifestyle. This process of assimilating this truth was challenging because my reluctance prevented me from understanding what my heart was truly struggling against. Despite difficulties and failures along the way, I was already practicing generosity and giving my tithes. These principles were instilled in my life from a young age when I learned under the teaching and care of my parents. This foundation helped me take my first steps—albeit hesitant— toward a deeper understanding of the true meaning of generosity.

I was still a minor and on my way to my first job. That day, I was excited, wearing the tie my father had given me so I could learn how to tie it for special occasions. I got on a crowded bus and about 20 minutes later got off at the stop that left me near the courthouse where I would begin my formal work life. On my way to the courthouse, I was caught in a sudden rainstorm and got soaked. Even so, I arrived at the expected time.

Upon arriving at my position, I noticed that my beautiful tie began to wrinkle and shrink as it dried. My emotional state was affected, but I maintained my 'pose'. That first day was intense. I focused my attention on work while at the same time tugging at my tie, stretching it and struggling with it. But that was okay; the day ended, and I put away my gift.

Tithing: More than a financial obligation

When I received my first paycheck after completing a month of work, my mother looked me straight in the eyes and said: *"Son, now that you've earned your money, don't forget to give God what belongs to Him."* She smiled and left me thinking. Although still somewhat reluctant and not fully understanding why, I joyfully gave, celebrating the opportunity and above all out of obedience while still thinking about what I would receive in return.

A Journey of learning

I rested because I saw an example at home and thought that if my parents gave their tithes and we could live as we did, I could also accept this challenge—even if it was just a decision of my soul. At that time, I believed that blessings were solely about financial results; in my innocence, I viewed it as a transaction: I gave to God and He returned it to me in prosperity. However, over time and as I practiced my faith, I discovered what I have been sharing with you in this book.

This experience taught me that giving tithe is not just a matter of finances, much less a biblical obligation; it is a decision of my heart and a search for a deeper relationship with God. I found that it is an act of worship and trust in God, who has always provided in all areas of my life. As human beings, I always strive to remember that by contributing, I am participating in something much greater than myself, aligning my heart with the teachings of the Word.

Tithing goes far beyond a financial transaction with God. It becomes a legitimate expression that reveals to me who is the Lord of all the areas in which I am involved. When we faithfully give the first fruits of our labor, we are declaring that He is the source of all our blessings and that we trust in this Provider.

Therefore, the giving of tithes should not be seen as an obligation, but as an opportunity for growth and spiritual maturity—it is undoubtedly a journey of self-discovery in how God honors our obedience and greatly blesses us. It is an act of worship and a clear testimony of total trust in God.

I don't need anything!

> *"The Eternal, my shepherd! I don't need anything. You put me in lush fields; you found calm waters, and from them, I can drink. Guided by your word, I regained strength and followed the right direction. Even if the road crosses the Valley of Death, I will not be afraid of anything, for you walk by my side. Your staff and rod give me security. You prepare a full dinner for me in front of my enemies. You renew me, and my discouragement disappears; my cup overflows with blessings. Your goodness and love chase after me every day of my life. So I will feel at home in the temple of God for all the time I live."* [Psalm 23 - The Message]

I love the translation of the Bible 'The Message,' especially Psalm 23. Some words used in this version really catch my attention, bringing an intense sense of peace. Knowing that I have the Provider taking care of every detail of my life gives me security at every step, whether I am awake or sleeping.

When we bless someone or give our part to the Lord, it's as if we are resting in God's presence, confident that He takes care of those He loves. This experience is like living through something up close, realizing that nothing more is needed besides divine richness, goodness, and love. It is a powerful reminder that, even in the most challenging stages, God's presence is enough to sustain us.

Feeling the presence of God

Feeling the presence of God is experiencing Him during any dilemma, whether prayers are answered or not. This presence I have experienced comes through the declaration of a believing heart—resting, grateful, and encouraged. That's why tithing and offerings, to me, are a clear condition of worship and of my love for Him. It is in this healthy relationship that I feel increasingly secure and convinced that I should never change what I do for the kingdom. This kind of giving can be extravagant and may shock those who have not lived or are not accustomed to a relationship at this level. The goodness and love that follow me justify the reminder that I don't need to yield to human limits, for I prefer to listen to what needs to and can happen.

Biblical examples of giving

Adam and Eve's sons, Abel and Cain, were confronted with life's realities. Cain had certainly heard the same words and had the same opportunities as his brother. However, he chose to follow his own plan. Abel, on the other hand, embraced the concept and pleased the heart of God by being obedient and choosing to give the necessary value and do what God expected.

Another example we see is Esau, who did not value the richness of his inheritance, while Jacob, his brother, seized the opportunity and took hold of the potential that his brother did not recognize. When we look at Abraham, it wasn't any different. Even having some internal questions about God's request, he respected it and proceeded with his mission, obeying to the point of offering his son Isaac as a sacrifice. But God stopped him in time, honoring his attitude. Ruth, for her part, gave herself to her mother-in-law Naomi, being recognized for her kindness and blessed by God. Her obedience and determination were rewarded with a completely unexpected future.

We read about the lives of the prophets, apostles, and teachers who gave their lives for the cause of Christ, obeying and fulfilling what they had in their hands to accomplish. And finally, our greatest example of giving: God offered us His best so that we could be transformed and receive Jesus!

An Inspiring Testimony

A Jiu-Jitsu professor, a training partner of mine, once gave me a testimony of his experience with money. At the time, although he was not converted, he would leave his wife at church but occasionally stop to listen to a sermon about tithing. Being intelligent as he was, he would listen and reflect on this divine mathematics. One day, he decided to "test" it and, to his surprise, it all worked out! In the same week he gave his tithe, something new happened, and he saw it was the hand of God. No matter who you are or where you are, when you apply the principle God has established, the principle of sowing and reaping will prove effective in your life. Remember, therefore, that it is up to us to take one more step in this process: *"Give with joy!"*

Divine Mathematics

I ask you: "If you give 10% of your income as a tithe to the church, how much is left for you?" Often, the answer comes with mockery: "Ninety percent, of course!" Others even look at me as if I were questioning their ability to do math. In human mathematics, it seems that 90% is left, but this view is deceptive. In fact, those ninety percent will be spent, and in the end, nothing will be left; you will consume it all! You will pay your bills, spend on food, and quickly satisfy your desires.

On the other hand, in divine mathematics, by giving the ten percent, what really remains? In the book When God Comes First, author Mike Hayes helps us understand that the first part—the 10%—is a sacrificial offering that must be made to see the multiplication of the rest. This is the reality of divine multiplication. The principle is established through a generous attitude. Not only are the ninety percent preserved, but the mercy and law of the Lord lead us to much more blessed paths. This is not a transaction with God; it is a sign of obedience and praise.

The difficulty and reluctance so many people encounter in this process is due to the need for a change in mindset. This transformation is not an easy process, especially when it comes to putting our hands on 'our' finances and delivering them by faith.

What's bad might get worse

Have you ever stopped to consider how much is truly lost daily due to unnecessary expenses? When analyzing our monthly expenses, we often realize how we have been robbed without realizing it. Simple situations, like a flat tire, repairing a refrigerator, or a lost investment, can significantly impact our budget. We are all exposed to these situations, and although God maintains dominion over all things, we still live under the influence of the prince of this world (Satan).

The Reality of the World

This world, controlled by forces that distort creation, subjects us to challenges and difficulties.

However, by recognizing the importance of prioritizing giving to God and practicing generosity, we can change our perspective and, consequently, our financial reality. Instead of being carried away by a scarcity mindset, we can embrace the abundance that comes from obedience and faith.

So, when we reflect on tithing and giving to God, we must understand that true wealth is not just in what is left over, but in the multiplication that occurs when we put God first. When we do this, we not only experience financial blessings, but also spiritual growth that transforms our lives. [Read Gen 3.17-18].

Jesus, the Prince of Peace, gave us a clear warning of what humanity would experience:

> *"I have said these things so that in me you may have peace. In this world you will have trouble, but take heart! I have overcome the world."*
> [John 16.33; read also 2 Corinthians 6.4-7]

The lie of humanism

You rely more on yourself and your own strength. One of the great deceptions of society is the almost generalized condition that man can "make it on his own", by his own ability alone and without God's help. In this case, the first justification regarding finances is: "I already know how to manage my money, and I don't need your advice"; "Can't you see that everything is going well?"; or, "What the Bible says may be good, but it doesn't fit in today's world; it's a thing of the past, the world has changed."

God himself established the times of blessing and the times of lack and drought. The seasons have been happening since the beginning of time, according to Genesis, when we read about creation. We also saw Joseph, at God's command, warning his king that he needed to be vigilant and look to the near future, giving him advice that wasn't just human; he was discerning a command from God. The advice was accepted, and there were seven years of plenty and another seven years of drought with much dryness in the land. The dryness spoiled and wiped out all the leftovers, affecting the economy of the surrounding kingdoms, except in the region that Joseph administered. Why? Because he listened to God and did as he had been instructed. As a result, they lived in abundance and had enough to lend, while others starved.

I've learned to call a situation like this a "margin". It's like the extra space on the page of a notebook where I make notes; it's the minutes I leave earlier and know will help me if I face a traffic jam; it's the reading, even if it's quick, but consistent, that makes me more knowledgeable about things; margin is the investment I make in life that will serve me when I need it, and it has to do with resources set aside for moments of urgency or unexpected need. The margin I build myself can be turned into profit.

And what is my role?

Distrust the integrity and character of the leader or the churches. It's true, the example we've seen in many organizations and churches is not encouraging and can take away from the person's pleasure in handing over finances to the Lord. I imagine that many people feed on these aspects and use them to back up their excuses and say: *"I'll take care of my money"*. Then I ask you: *"Does this money really belong to you?"* After all, what is my role in building this legacy? Well, I already know that if I keep or use what isn't mine, we call it stealing. The truth here is: will you believe in the norms of the Word, or will you act like the majority: *"my way"*?

When I say that I only do what is my way, I give room for individualistic and selfish ideas. For example, if I see a thief in action, no matter how much it scares me, I can't generalize and point out that all people are bad and, therefore, I don't trust anyone because they might steal from me? We look at the governments of nations where there are people who corrupt themselves and take advantage of the opportunities they must defraud and seek their wealth. But is it fair to say that we don't need government or its services? Nor can I say that every government or every person in public service acts dishonestly. Can we no longer believe and live as righteous people, doing the right thing even when others walk against the law? If we see a judge making a lot of mistakes in a soccer match, can we say that all judges are bad? Obviously not.

It's true, not all men value honesty, not all doctors operate with zeal for life and many judges or pastors don't walk in a fair and consistent way. Even so, we can't say that we don't need them. I don't believe that all doctors, pastors and other professionals are doing and living wrong just because I know some who are corrupt! In the same way, we need to believe in and fight for a healthy and holy church. So, I try to do and spread what is my part, seeking to have clean hands and a pure heart, as well as not agreeing with arbitrariness, in the struggle to produce something better.

May we then reflect on these principles and apply divine mathematics to our lives. When we give our tithes and offerings, we are not just fulfilling an obligation, but investing in a deep relationship with God, who will always repay us with blessings beyond what we can imagine.

Provision and Prosperity

It took me a while to understand that a rich person is different from a person who prospers. My speeches and what I'm used to hearing need to pass through the sieve of decency and theological order. A phrase like: *"When you give to God, He will make you rich!"* amazes me, because something like that can become a springboard of danger for the innocent heart of a person seeking God's justice. Just because the "anointed one" speaks from the pulpit doesn't mean that it comes from God.

Without wishing to disrespect the men and women God has chosen to minister, the church is the headquarters where the rules and precepts that can lead people to higher flights must be observed with great fear. Even so, it seems that the zeal for the purity of the Gospel has been lost, and we see leaders who move away and seem to pretend not to value the conservative character of the Word.

Personally, I don't embrace every kind of gospel proclaimed in many places, because a lot of human invention has confused people's hearts. I prefer to stick to biblical messages that are contextualized and presented with coherence and ethics. One of them is the certainty that the sower sows his seed in the ground and must expect his harvest to be abundant. He must work and always do his best, because times are bad, and we always need the Lord's grace.

The Falacy of the Prosperity Gospel

The problem with the prosperity gospel is that it emphasizes reward and not motivation, because God blesses giving with the right heart! And if this prosperity gospel is dangerous, there is another one that is associated with messages about finances and becomes just as destructive, which is the gospel that works on the soul and generates the fear of poverty and scarcity. They say: *"If you don't take advantage of this moment - with this seed - you could miss out on the multiplication that awaits you!"*. Yes, the sower plants and waits for his harvest, but is that the seed you are presenting to me? What else am I hearing from God and what else is the Word instructing me on this subject?

Both gospels mentioned have been preached and they are very dangerous. The true gospel presents the constant provision and blessing! The Provider God knows that my fruit serves as a blessing for someone else and for the kingdom of God, and that my giving adjusts my heart within the actions I am involved in. So tithing was a great place to start, because it has always been a decision of obedience and faith from my will.

The truth about tithing

If you still don't tithe, you need to understand that this doesn't make you a bad person, someone with a bad heart who doesn't love God any less than someone else. The devil is always looking for a heart to lead astray, because he likes to whisper lies in people's ears. It's also possible that you haven't yet discovered what it means to have a generous and willing heart.

The truth is that many of us are still growing in our understanding. Some say: "I'd love to give my tithe, but I can't!". That person is just afraid to take the first step of faith, because money has been their security all their life. In church, and I hope in yours too, we are taught that we can only find security in the Word of God.

Meditate on the following text for yourself:

> *"Remember: he who sows little will also reap little, and he who sows bountifully will also reap bountifully. Each one should give as he has determined in his heart, not with regret or out of obligation, for God loves a cheerful giver. And God is able to make all grace abound toward you, so that in all things, at all times, having everything you need, you may abound in every good work. As it is written: 'He distributed, he gave his goods to the needy; his righteousness endures forever. He who supplies seed to the sower and bread to the eater will also supply you and multiply the seed and make the fruits of his righteousness grow. You will be enriched in every way, so that you can be generous at all times...'"* [2Corinthians 9:6-15]

The law of sowing and tithing in the New Testament

The law of sowing, as discussed in 2 Corinthians 8 and 9, deals with the contribution. Many pastors separate the topics of first fruits and tithes from contributions. The contribution mentioned by Paul refers to a specific collection for the brethren in Judea (Jerusalem), who had been facing a financial crisis since the time of Acts 2.

When we read Galatians, the issue of tithing becomes more transparent, but still needs understanding. Although tithing was not established in the Old Testament Law as a curse, but rather as a demonstration of priority in the will of the human heart, Christ resolved this issue once and for all. The victory, success and joy that we all seek come through faith alone.

Therefore, the practice of tithing is not necessarily an obligation on the part of the believer, but a way of demonstrating the primacy of the Lord and evidence that he is willing, without the ties of the world, to recognize God as Lord in worship.

Christ's Redemption

"Christ redeemed us from the curse of the Law when he became a curse in our place, for it is written, 'Cursed is everyone who is hung on a tree. ' This was so that in Christ Jesus the blessing of Abraham might also come to the Gentiles, that we might receive the promise of the Spirit through faith." [Galatians 3:13-14]

God has never been the author of curses, even though we live in a world of curses. However, just as it was for God's children in the past, there is a condition in place: He always waits for my decision and my step of faith. It is my decision to establish

Him as First in my life, so that I can enjoy all that is already available and promised.

The importance of intention

In the New Testament, the idea of tithing is more closely linked to evidence of worshipping the Lord. The seriousness of this matter is emphasized by Jesus, who said to his disciples and the Pharisees:

"For I tell you, unless your righteousness is far superior to that of the Pharisees and teachers of the law, you will by no means enter the kingdom of heaven." [Matthew 5:20]

He also warned:

"Woe to you, teachers of the law and Pharisees, hypocrites! You tithe mint, dill and cumin, but you have neglected the most important precepts of the law: justice, mercy and faithfulness. You must practice these things, without omitting those." [Matthew 23:23]

Jesus highlighted the importance of the intention behind the offering when referring to the widow's contribution:

> *"Jesus looked and saw the rich putting their contributions into the offering boxes. He also saw a poor widow putting in two small copper coins. And he said, 'I tell you, this poor widow has put in more than all the others. All these gave of what they had left; but she, out of her poverty, gave all that she had to live on.'"* [Luke 21:1-4]

This passage teaches us that, although we can contribute when we have money left over in our budget, when we give back what is the Lord's, we must do so from the start, with a generous heart. Jesus appreciated the widow's offering, who gave not silver or gold coins, but copper. This shows us that God wants to receive everything that is in our hearts, not just the leftovers of our work.

Thus, true contribution is not measured only by material value, but by intention and commitment. By understanding the importance of sowing and generosity, we can align our actions with the principles of worship and love for God, reflecting the true essence of what it means to be a true giver.

The need for financial education

If I want to train my body in a gym, I need to get up from the sofa and sweat, sweat a lot to lose a few kilos and stay physically regenerated. It won't work if I just pay the monthly fee. So, understand my statement: *"You'll never be able to tithe until you start!"*.

The standard way sustained for centuries within Christian organizations shows us that there is much more incentive in classes that work on the soul and spirit of their members, using the teachings of the prophets, the psalms of David, the parables of Jesus and the whole context of Paul's journeys. However, little is said about personal finance and the principles that govern a life of financial success, which can lead a person to a solid understanding of how to build a differentiated life in their place of work.

May we reflect on the importance of understanding God's provision and the true prosperity he offers. When we give our tithes and offerings, we are not just fulfilling an obligation, but investing in a deep relationship with God, who will always repay us with blessings beyond what we can imagine. Let's seek true wisdom and discernment in our finances, aligning our actions with divine principles that will guide us to an abundant and purposeful life.

"On the first day of the week, let each one of you set aside at home according to his prosperity, and gather, so that collections may not be made when I come." [1 Corinthians 16:2]

<u>Reflection 1</u>

You come to me and say: "Mark, I hear you won't be in town next week. My car is at the mechanics, and I need to work, I must go to various places. Can I use your car on those days?" I replied: "Of course you can! The key and the document are here! Even the gas tank is full. You can use it all you want."

A few days go by, and you knock on my door again, saying: "My wife and I prayed and felt it in our hearts to give you this car!" I laugh and reply: "Did you hit your head somewhere? It's my car!" You were just bringing back what is mine. I paid for the car, serviced it, filled up the gas tank and handed over the key and the document so that you wouldn't have any problems if someone doubted it.

The parallel with God

This parallel applies perfectly to the things of God, especially when we talk about tithing. "If you take your step of faith and return what is mine from the beginning, then I will bless you in ways you cannot imagine." Regardless of what the world says and how people present it, the point here is not just about financial return; it involves character and the will to do what is right. Those who work hard and intelligently will earn a lot of money; and the blessing of recognition and obedience extends to the whole family, your business, health, relationships, marriage, ministry and everything else that is related to your purpose in life. You will enjoy your harvest always and abundantly when you surrender what is rightfully His.

Reflection 2

Responsibility and Tithing: A Necessary Parallel. Imagine that you are my boss in a company where I work every day. You trust me completely; I try to be an honest person; I respect my coworkers and I'm seen as someone with integrity. Today is Friday and, after lunch, you call me and say: "This amount I entrust to you, but first separate this percentage and pay the company's water bill and energy bill. The rest is yours, because of your excellent work. Congratulations!"

The lack of responsibility

As it's already Friday, I'm rushing around, but I still don't have time to do everything I should. I go home and think: "I'll pay on Monday." The weekend passes and I end up using that "extra" money for other things. Two months go by and suddenly the water and electricity service is cut off at the company. You investigate and realize that the bills have not been paid. After a quick search, you discover that I was responsible!

Now, what would you say?

- I got what was mine.
- I also received what didn't belong to me.
- I didn't value the money I was responsible for.
- I acted like a thief.
- I wasn't responsible for paying it back and I used the rest without authorization.
- The company made a loss because of my irresponsibility.
- I didn't do my part.
- Is this person of integrity, recognized even by my friends, a reality?
- What other consequences could there be because of this act?

The parallel with tithes

This example leads us to a parallel with millions of people who, without realizing it, do the same with their tithes. If I act in this way, at some point I will realize it and suffer similar damage and consequences. And even worse, whenever someone fails to do the right thing, the result of that mistake can affect other people around them. Cases like these make us wonder if many evangelical churches and organizations wouldn't be stronger and have a greater reach in their work if they didn't have to deal with similar situations.

The relevance expected from their projects can be diminished by the irresponsibility of many. All this generates consequences for the spirit, soul and body, becoming a disservice that occurs because most Christians do not identify their gain as an undeserved gift and opportunity.

The illusion of self-sufficiency

The human tendency is to believe that you don't need help to negotiate what is yours and, consequently, to believe that you can manage what doesn't belong to you. The result is visible in everyday life, where people suffer, trapped in their problems, many of which are generated from doors opened by forgetfulness - or ignorance. Lack of commitment not only has financial consequences, but also manifests itself physically, in relationships and through so many other losses that could have been avoided.

Therefore, as we reflect on our responsibility with tithes and offerings, it is essential that we recognize that each act of giving is an opportunity to honor God and take care of what He has entrusted to us. May we be diligent and responsible, understanding that the way we handle our finances is not just a practical matter, but a reflection of our character and faith. So, when we give our tithes, we are not only fulfilling an obligation, but also investing in a deep relationship with God, who will always repay us with blessings beyond what we can imagine.

Reflection 3

I have a memory that fills me with joy when I recall a significant change we made in our church. We had been looking for a new space for some time and when we finally found a building much larger than our current one, we were able to sign a contract that would comfortably accommodate our audience and fit in with what we were willing to pay in rent.

The church in action

The reaction of the members was spectacular and suddenly everyone began to wholeheartedly express their offers of time, physical strength, money and skills. The building was rented just a few days before the end-of-year celebrations, a challenging time to make any changes that weren't in the lens of Christmas. Of course, this is a time when people get busy with parties, focus their attention on family, travel and meetings with professional friends.

However, the move left us with no options, and the most economical decision was to give up the old building and move quickly into the new one. We were confident and nothing could divert our attention. We realized that many of the messages and words that had been sown were now sprouting in each person's heart. The new space was more than we had imagined.

The challenge of transformation

We received the space completely empty, like a large warehouse, without walls or any partitions. We needed to tidy everything up, create a suitable layout and accommodate our members and children as soon as they returned from their holidays.

With everyone working together, in just over two weeks we were ready to move in and worship God comfortably.

Builders, painters, financial donations, willing people carrying weights and cleaning up the remains of the work - it all came together perfectly! We saw the contagious happiness of offering our first fruits of time and care to the Lord.

The firstfruits in action

The people's demonstration was powerful when put into action. To this day, few times have we seen the church's finances as robust as in the first few months after the move.

This experience taught us that when we unite around a common purpose and hand over what we have to God, not only will we have provision, but we can also be surprised by abundant blessings. It's always good to remember that every act of generosity and every step of faith can be the seeds that, when planted in the fertile soil of God's kingdom, can produce extraordinary fruit, even if unexpected.

"Honor the Lord with your possessions, and with the firstfruits of all your increase; and your barns shall be filled with plenty, and your winepresses shall overflow with wine." [Proverbs 3.9-10]

"You shall bring the firstfruits of the first fruits of your land into the house of the Lord your God." [Exodus 23.19a]

The first fruits are basically the beginning of a loving relationship with the Father. It's our first act of faith before something new is given to us; it's a way of getting to know our heart better. For example, the first salary from a new job, the first fruit from a crop, the first animals from a farm, the first result from a business transaction, etc. Of course, like all the acts we've discussed, the firstfruit is a voluntary act given from the heart. The firstfruits is the giving of my first part of what I have received and represents the first fruits of a new phase. The offering of the firstfruits is the sanctification of the rest of my income and is the consecration I make to God, believing that He will multiply, as He wishes, all the rest. How can this be calculated? Simple: it's the value of a day's work at the end of a month, for example.

It's good to know that some scholars differ in their understanding of the firstfruits, explaining that they are no longer relevant to our day. However, they are frequently quoted in the New Testament. I respect those who think differently, and there shouldn't be any discussion on this subject, since it's about the willing, generous and available heart before God. Even though there is no mention of obligation, the New Testament did not abolish the Law of Firstfruits:

> *"If the firstfruits are holy, so is the dough; and if the root is holy, so are the branches."*
> [Romans 11.16]

Professor and teacher Luciano Subirá talks about the Law of Firstfruits: "In mentioning the need to give honor to the Lord in our finances, the Word of the Lord talks about our possessions and the firstfruits of our income. It's not just about honoring Him with our possessions, nor is it about honoring Him only with our income, but with the first fruits of that income."

The Aurélio Dictionary's definition of first fruits is: "First fruits; first productions; first effects; first profits; first feelings; first enjoyments; beginnings, preludes." The biblical definition is no different. Behind a whole doctrine based on explicit teachings and implicit figures, the Scriptures show us the importance that God gives to our act of giving Him our first fruits, the definition of which is: "the first part of something."

God didn't institute offerings because he needed them, but to test our hearts in one of the areas where we show great attachment. It's no different with the Law of First Fruits. God doesn't need the first fruits. We are the ones who need Him first in our lives, and this is an excellent exercise to keep our hearts aware of that.

So, all we have to do is practice and reap the fruits of our obedience.

"But each one in his own order: Christ the firstfruits, then those who are Christ's at his coming." [1 Corinthians 15:23]

Jesus is the firstfruits of the Father who was given to us so that we could, through this act, be blessed and multiplied in the grace he has given us. Remember, do everything as an act of love and faith, recognizing that by honoring God with what you have, you will open the door to a life of abundance and blessings.

Firstfruits is a return of thanks from the heart, which we give to God where we are nourished and instructed by the Word of God. If we keep our first fruits, we don't have the opportunity to see the seeds multiply in the course of our work, function, business, etc. Giving the first fruits, as well as tithes and offerings, are ways of acknowledging God first. Leaving it until last means not giving Him first place. Firstfruits is putting God and the faith we have in the right place at the right time.

Do a search on your computer or cell phone and you'll find much more on this subject. Allow yourself to work on and exhaust this subject by doing your research and listening to what God says in your heart. This means working on your paradigms, giving the Holy Spirit freedom to speak and rebuilding in you and through you an altar of worship to the Lord - don't forget who you are: a temple of the Holy Spirit.

The transformation you surely seek and hope for comes through the renewal of your understanding.

"Do not imitate the behavior and customs of this world, but let God transform you by changing your way of thinking, so that you may experience God's good, pleasing and perfect will for you" [Romans 12.2].

The Transforming Power of Offerings

The act of giving is a blessing demonstration of love that resonates with many people. We see it happening in all forms and in all walks of life; whether a Christian or not, everyone loves to feel that they are blessing others.

We learn from each other, and this demonstration of affection and love has been passed down through the centuries, as we've already said, reaching us. The joy of handing over a birthday present, the simple gesture of blessing someone who is hungry next to you, a charity meeting or a specific need that you perceive and that makes your heart move to give - these are all opportunities to express generosity.

The more open I am to kindness like this, the more my heart fills with joy. It's a transforming experience that not only touches the lives of those who receive, but also enriches the lives of those who give.

Even better is knowing that God is pleased with this personal selflessness. He was the one who gave his only Son, an act of immeasurable love. That's why, in the next chapter, I'll talk about the Five Jars, a concept I learned from teacher and master Craig Hill.

It's not just the will or the fact that I have an open heart that drives me to give. It is essential that I prepare myself so that my actions are increasingly constant and responsible, both towards myself, my family and the church where I give my time, skills and financial resources. Every gesture of generosity is an opportunity to sow love and blessings. In doing so, we not only fulfill a spiritual principle, but we also become instruments of transformation in the lives of others and in our own lives. May we always be open to giving, knowing that each offering is an expression of our love and gratitude to God.

Our Responsibility

- It's about giving, yes!
- It is to help, yes!
- It is to share, yes!
- It's a decision, yes!

Living this truth is a decision, recognizing that the joy of giving is an expression of our love and gratitude to God.

"But seek first his kingdom and his righteousness, and all these things will be added to you." [Matthew 6.33]

172

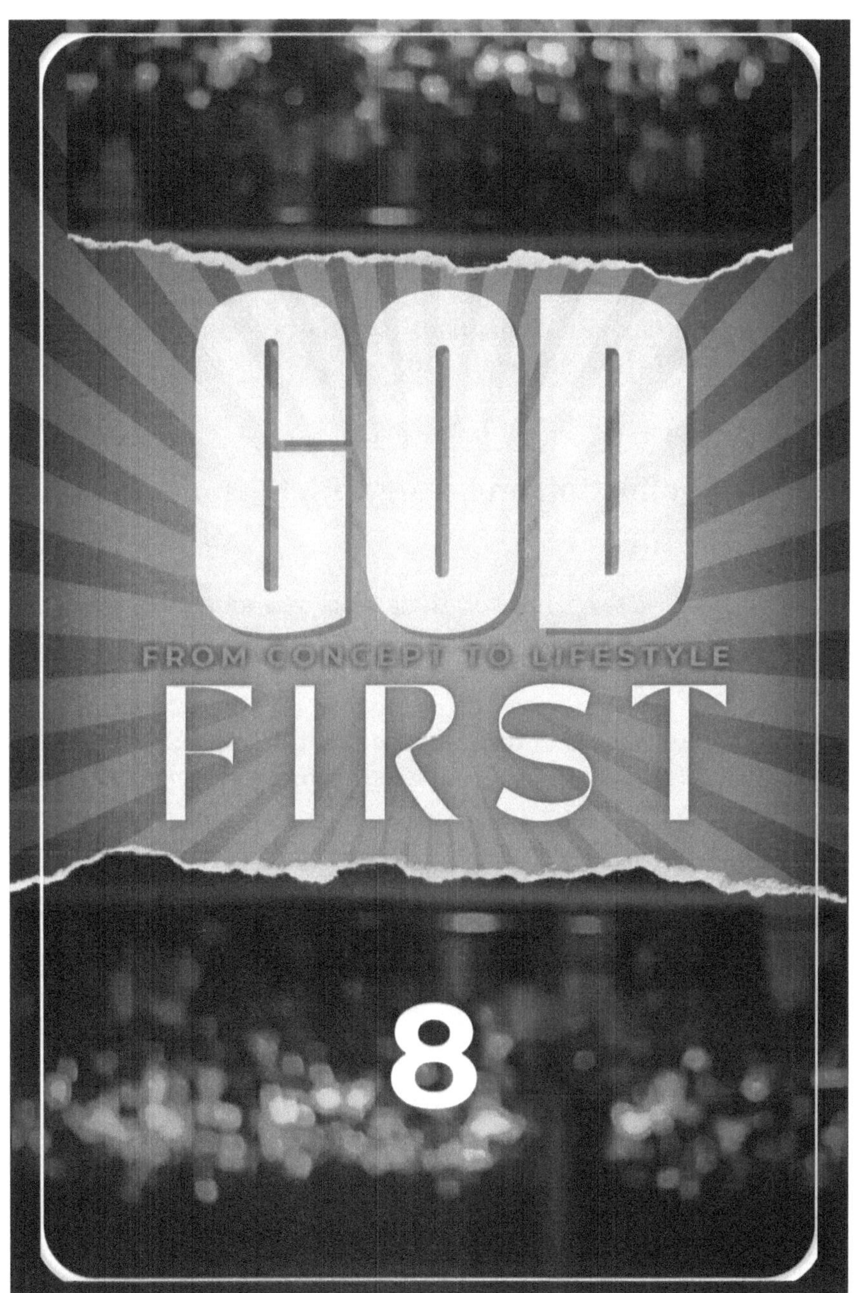

GOD
FROM CONCEPT TO LIFESTYLE
FIRST
8

"But God has revealed it to us through the Spirit. The Spirit searches all things, even the deepest things of God." [1Corinthians 2:10]

Reflection on Living with Purpose

I used to spend everything I received, emptying my bank balance and hoping that something would change the next day. Over time, I realized that many who were struggling to survive settled into the same unfortunate strategy. This rollercoaster of desires and expectations, however, goes against everything we learn about God from His Word. Situations and habits of this kind heighten our anxiety and worries. A few years ago, I realized that this behavior could be transformed not only in my life and that of my family, but also in the lives of my brothers and sisters and everyone I could reach.

The Road to Transformation

To change this short-term mentality, I had to give time to time and train my mind, but above all my heart. We learn from the Word that we don't wake up every day just to survive the experiences we will have, but to walk as the winners we really are. Neither you nor I should live as survivors in a frightened society. Remember: The Church is victorious! That's why we can't negotiate what Jesus Christ has already guaranteed: we are more than conquerors. This truth must be non-negotiable within us.

Discovering Purpose and Values

To get out of 'survivor' mode and into 'more than winner' mode, it is essential to follow some guidelines, especially for those who believe in Jesus' teachings and seek the Lord with all their heart. If you consider yourself a winner, you must not accept living as a survivor. It is essential to discover your purpose and values, nurturing the desire to share all that you have received with others.

The prosperity I share with my family today is the result of obedience and focus on God's purposes for our home. Humanly speaking, we always face challenges and obstacles, but everything I do is with the aim of getting to know God better and ensuring that He comes first in my life. He is God First, and my lifestyle commits to this truth at every step.

I can't attribute my progress to myself or anyone else; humanity, no matter how much it tries to solve its moral and integrity problems, still owes God everything he has already done for us. And, above all, we don't deserve the price that was paid on the cross.

Are you ready? Then let's go!

Come with me...

With that, I want you to get ready, because you will discover a recipe - among many that the Word of God presents - that will establish you with financial prosperity: without tricks, without major emotions, without putting your life and career at risk and without religiosity. The result and the future that awaits you will depend solely and exclusively on a commitment to yourself. But first, I need to remind you a little of the biblical story of King Solomon.

In this short story, I want you to focus your attention on a few points that can underpin your whole life. David, as Solomon's father, had established a path of blessing for his generation, just as I seek it for mine, and you too must work for it. Another point is that absolutely all of Solomon's prosperity came from a request that apparently wasn't connected to riches and money. When asked by God about his request, he focused on the wisdom he wanted to obtain. This obviously didn't take God by surprise, but because he saw Solomon's pure heart, he offered much more. Solomon asked God for wisdom. This was granted to him, and he became one of the most prosperous men on earth, the wisest among men, just in his decisions, until he lost himself in his human weaknesses.

Solomon's Fall and Its Lessons

In 1 Kings, King Solomon, despite all the wealth that surrounded him, faced a weakness that led him to be out of control with women, resulting in his downfall. He had Egyptian, Moabite, Idumean, Sidonian and Hittite women available in his palace, totaling 700 wives and 300 concubines. A friend of mine commented on this: "Instead of icing on the cake, lime dust!" This phrase sums up the irony of Solomon's situation. He had everything going for him, but he chose pleasure. Even though he was wise before men, he didn't understand true prosperity.

Solomon let himself be carried away by what his eyes desired, and his love for all those women corrupted his heart. The central point is the luxury of being carried away by human passions, leading him to do what was evil in the eyes of the Lord.

The Quest for Prosperity and its pitfalls

In our quest for prosperity, we often focus on possessions, positions and knowledge. We value our passions to the point of celebrating a sporting victory more than the very presence of God, who is the reason for our living. It's easy to observe this behavior among people, especially in the country of soccer. We jump, shout, cheer and feel sad when our team loses. But what about God?

We should reflect on how we balance our priorities and remember that true victory lies in recognizing and celebrating God's presence in our lives.

Without realizing it, we fall into the same traps and ruin as those who don't have God. Solomon's neglect provoked God's indignation, because he transgressed the statutes and laws of the Almighty, forgetting who had really provided him with everything he had.

Solomon's neglect brought division to the nation of Israel, a powerful reminder that our choices have consequences. By divine mercy, the kingdom was not destroyed, but this story teaches us a valuable lesson: for the sake of the God you serve, seek a full and worthy relationship with the Creator. He is the one who can truly bless you, if you obey Him.

It is wrong and incomprehensible to want to customize faith, adapting it to personal interests. Solomon's story shows us that we can choose to prioritize the wisdom that comes from God in our lives or, like him, distract ourselves with what is not a priority, feasting on the desires of the soul until we fall into disgrace.

When we put God first, He guides us away from distractions, leading us on a path of true prosperity that encompasses all areas of life, including the spiritual and emotional. May our journey be marked by obedience and the desire to glorify God in everything we do. In doing so, we will find lasting purpose and a peace that transcends circumstances.

The warning about the false teachers

In John 10:10, we learn that *"the thief comes only to steal and kill and destroy; I have come that they may have life and have it to the full."*

For many years, we have been taught and believed that "the thief" refers to the devil. However, many teachers of the Word suggest that the thief represents the false teachers - pastors, prophets and evangelists or anyone who cares only about rewards, and not about the welfare of the sheep. These deceivers come with strategies ready to exploit the innocent, perpetuating a cycle of deception that is not new.

Solomon's story teaches us that true wealth and happiness do not lie in possessions or achievements, but in a genuine relationship with God. By prioritizing divine wisdom and obedience, we can avoid the traps that led Solomon to ruin and instead live an abundant life, as promised by Christ.

In my universe of life, when observing relationships between people, it is common to notice at least two types of mentality in the way business and money are conducted. Often, people develop their lives and businesses by choosing between a limited mindset or a prosperous mindset.

The limited mindset and its effects

People with a limited mindset often take 100% ownership of their earnings, focusing only on themselves or, at most, their immediate family. This behavior is the starting point for our reflection. Their investments, businesses and lifestyles often revolve around fear of the future or preoccupation with the present, living with the dread - or even fear - of loss.

People like this don't learn from the past and end up repeating their choices, even those that clearly weren't beneficial. This limited mindset may not be a conscious decision; it is often fueled by a lack of confidence in their ability to keep what they have achieved and a fear of what the future may bring.

It's crucial to recognize that this way of thinking can restrict our potential and limit opportunities for growth. By developing a more open and trusting mindset, we can transform our relationship with money and possessions, allowing new possibilities to reveal themselves along the way.

The prosperous mindset and its opportunities

On the other hand, we find fewer people willing to open themselves up to a range of opportunities by adopting a prosperous mindset. These people often show a willingness to limit their spending and, in a controlled way, discern how to use their income. In addition, they are open to sharing their earnings with others, recognizing the value of generosity.

It's important to note that we shouldn't just label people by what we see or what we assume. I'm talking about apparent habits and an unscientific perception. However, the application of these two mentalities is deeply linked to the individual understanding that each person develops throughout their process of maturity, whether inside or outside the churches. Much of what we learn about life and money is shaped by living with our parents, our culture, the friendships we cultivate and the circumstances that surround us as we grow into adults.

Unfortunately, there has been little emphasis on resource generation and career development in churches. There is significant concern about keeping contributions coming in, but there is often a failure to "teach the child in the way" when it comes to saving and individual financial growth. It is essential that faith communities address these issues, empowering their members to thrive holistically in all areas of their lives.

The path to success

Everyone in the world can - and should - work towards success in all areas of life. However, I emphasize once again, any security you seek cannot be based solely on wealth or human knowledge. That would be like building a castle on sand. True security has a name: JESUS, the way, the truth and the life.

Each person has a task to fulfill. I want to look back one day and say the same words as Jesus, when he saw that his work had been accomplished as the Father expected. May we then choose the prosperous mindset, trusting in God and His provision, as we work to fulfill our purpose and impact the lives of others around us. Jesus gave his testimony of what had been placed in his hands:

The University of the Family and its impact

The Family University, founded more than 25 years ago by Jorge Nishimura, began as a personal effort and today has thousands of volunteers spread throughout Brazil. This institution stands out for offering valuable teachings through great teachers and specialists in the most diverse areas of biblical teaching. One of the outstanding teachers is Dr. Craig Hill, a long-time friend of mine, whom I have had the privilege of interpreting for on several occasions.

Dr. Craig is not only a Master of Communication and the art of marriage relationships, but also an investor in the financial market. He shares in-depth knowledge about the secrets of finance and how we can prosper using the fruits of our labor. Importantly, regardless of income, there is always room for multiplication.

During one of his lectures, something caught my attention. As I listened to him, his words organized themselves in my mind like a map, especially when he mentioned "The Five Jars", a concept that is also covered in his book "Five Secrets of Wealth". Many of us, especially within churches, have never received proper instruction on finances. When we look at history, we realize that many important teachings have remained hidden for centuries, overshadowed by human systems that distort clear thinking. As a result, millions of people do not know how to develop or plan their savings and acquisitions, often for lack of knowledge.

"My people are being destroyed because they lack knowledge." [Hosea 4.6]

It is essential that institutions like the Family University continue to address these issues, empowering people to make informed financial decisions and prosper in all areas of their lives.

Discussion on personal finance

Despite the difficulties I faced when learning about personal finance, I am grateful to see that this topic is no longer taboo among Christians. Today, finances are discussed in a more direct and transparent way, and even better when they respect biblical principles. When approached correctly, this subject offers the opportunity for all of God's children to be blessed by the reward of their work.

The Five Jars of provision

I would like to explore the concept of the Five Jars of Provision by illustrating it with a conversation between a father and son. From an early age, the boy is taught about financial fundamentals and, over time, becomes a financially successful person among his friends in the neighborhood and at school. When he comes of age, he manages to buy his house in cash, the result of putting into practice everything he learned from his father. This son received from him a solid understanding of finances, as well as the importance of cultivating a healthy relationship with God. He was inspired by his father's teachings and applied the principles of generosity and financial wisdom to his life, building a legacy of prosperity and faith.

"The poor are dominated by the rich; whoever borrows is in their hands." [Proverbs 22.7]

"When people cannot see what God is doing, they stumble over themselves; but when they pay attention to what he reveals, they are the most blessed." [Proverbs 29.18]

Overcoming challenges in difficult times

2020 was one of the most challenging years in our house. We have faced great struggles, lost loved ones during the pandemic and watched companies close their doors, leaving many people completely upset and afraid. What could have been catastrophic for us, however, turned into days full of blessings, because we were already practicing the principles I teach in this book with obedience. We faced the circumstances, sought strength in God and, because we weren't taken by surprise, we managed to win each fight, one at a time.

A blessed victory

That year ended, and today we can say that, despite the circumstances and the loss of many loved ones, it was also a time when we could count and testify to the Lord's blessings. We had been living in the same place for more than ten years, renting an apartment, and we were getting ready to start building our dream house.

We understood that God's plans come before our own, and by doing our part, that is:

- consistently bringing our share - the tithes - to God what belongs to him,

- Offering towards people and projects that bless,

- Setting aside savings for difficult times and,

- Saving to invest in our dreams.

We were immensely blessed. This experience taught us that, even during challenges, faith and obedience can lead us to significant victories. Thanks to this, during the crisis we managed to pay all our bills on time. Everything we prepared, at the right time, God opened the doors and introduced us to the people who were part of this victory. Before the year was out, we had already sold the land and bought the place where we live today in cash, as well as renovating every square meter of this wonderful home that we won by God's grace - and by the effort we made not to lose sight of practicing this excellent tool.

The path of persistence

What happened didn't come for free, without effort or determination. We were the ones who sought and prepared, with the grace and choice to obey what the Word teaches us. Other dreams are already underway, and we will certainly see them come to fruition, each in its own time and according to the Father's will.

In the same way, it will happen to you if you just persist to the end. May we all commit to following these principles and trusting in God's providence, knowing that He is faithful to fulfill His promises in our lives.

The importance of Financial Planning

See that I'm dealing with the basis and foundations of tithing; later, I'll talk about how to do it. When I talk about obedience, surrender and determination, these behaviors involve a person's entire being. I need to know where I am to assess how and how far I can go. If I want to lose weight but I have no idea how much fat I need to burn, I can remain in the realm of guesswork. Through trial and error, I manage to do something, but it will happen without much responsibility. And without having an objective and a goal of how much I need to achieve, everything will become a bit hazy and purposeless. The same applies to my time - I must know how much and when to use it for important, urgent or circumstantial things.

Using these premises, it's easier to see when other people don't value the input of their finances enough. At home, we have learned to discover the path of the money that comes into our hands. Today, more than ever, we ask ourselves the following question:

- "Do we realize how much we have brought to God with our tithes of thanksgiving and worship?";

- "What part of our finances do we give to people in need?";

- "What have I done with my savings, how are my investments and businesses?";

- "Am I up to date with the Lord or am I playing at being a believer?".

It's questions like these that, if not dealt with seriously, can repeatedly lead a person back to square one and depend on unpleasant restarts. But if adjustments are made and treated with the necessary urgency, observing the required maintenance, everything will become clearer.

Again, on this journey to financial 'health', it is necessary to know the path of your money, which involves taking safe, consistent and conscious steps. Time will pass, there will be effort and hard work, but in the generous moments of celebration or of greater financial instability in the market, this security and preparation will serve as an anchor and produce the desired rest.

Living God First

I want you to look very seriously at this last argument and, without question, fully grasp the concept of what it means to live God First. Only then will you be able to experience it as a lifestyle and as something definitive and necessary for your whole life. If you are already someone who has a well-adjusted financial life, who consistently builds, rents, saves, invests or travels, congratulations on having done your homework. Conceptually, there's nothing wrong with that, and there's nothing more pleasant than reaping the rewards of your investments generated with honesty and hard work.

However, the fundamental aspect of abundance is not having things or even being rich, but living in peace with oneself and, above all, with God. Here's the question again: "Has God been first in my life? Have I given him back everything that isn't mine?". May we live this truth, giving our tithe with joy and trust in God, our Provider and Intimate Friend, who will never let us fall short.

To correctly gauge a person's behavior and commitment to their finances, there are many points that can be discussed. When it comes to handing over to God what is His, you or I will certainly present our truths and concepts, which could lead to a long and exhausting discussion. But for our conversation to be more objective, and before we go into the practice of these concepts, I want to present five aspects, which I believe serve as a light in the darkness of human doubts and questions. When someone delves into the subject of finance, these aspects are usually raised:

<u>Aspect One</u> – Do you have a purpose?

It's possible that you don't know the real purpose of giving. Remember what we've been discussing: we err through ignorance - because we don't know the truth - and we err when we forget or don't give due value to what has been shared with us. This is a good time to reflect on how much you still need to achieve a deeper understanding. Evaluate your heart: what have you been listening to or watching that has really become a treasure trove, and so you doubt everything? The best thing to do after learning something new, even if you haven't fully grasped it, is to repeat it and practice it consistently.

I once attended a sermon by Miles Monroe, who made a very important point about the time we have and the choices we make every day. He reminded us that every morning, each person wakes up with the same amount of value: 24 hours. Each hour of the day can be seen as a monetary unit, our investment currency. So, when you wake up, you have a wealth of 24 coins. However, at the end of the day, each person ends up with a different amount, depending on how they spent or invested their coins over the last 24 hours.

If you're an intelligent person, you've used your coins wisely, investing more time reading a book, attending a lecture or studying about subjects that interest you and make you grow. Each 'coin' has been used to acquire knowledge about your work and for intellectual or spiritual development.

The truth is, however, that nobody wakes up smart, says the preacher. It takes practice, hard work and commitment. Therefore, if a person is less intelligent and ignores the things of God, they will lack determination and will inevitably exchange what is good for the superficial things that their soul desires.

It's sad to say, but: "If you act like that, that's all you'll ever achieve!" It's true that what you exchange your time for is what you become. Every hour is worth what you gain or lose. You buy life with the investment of your time. If you want to change the quality of the life you lead, you will need to change the way you invest your time, and your lifestyle will need to undergo a complete restructuring.

<u>Aspect Two</u> – Learn Divine Mathematics

Pay attention to this statement: even if you haven't truly believed, when you give God what is His, you will always receive more than you invested. Our math has been very "dumb" over the years, because we believe that we can do math and business with God, as we do in the world in normal situations. We only think and evaluate the present, measure everything and act according to what we see and what fits into our accounts. Our soul is like that, and walks according to our anxieties, desires and passions.

One of the biggest mistakes we all make is not realizing that God owes nothing to anyone! The best result of these mathematical calculations is when we realize that we will always be in debt for what has already been consummated on the cross. There is absolutely nothing we can do that will benefit us in any way.

From decision to action!

For real success to happen and for you to have consistency in advancing and multiplying your earnings, the Five Jars tool - which we'll come to shortly - needs to be considered seriously. If you use money in the same way as most people, i.e. without proper planning, it's very likely that your savings will be used up by the end of the day. That's why a prosperous mindset must be part of your identity!

I believe that your mindset has already been transformed and that you have accepted the challenge of obedience and faith. You have humbled yourself before God for the mistakes of the past and you want to use the Five Jars tool to realize what you have always dreamed of and which has been echoing within you, now restored. When this happens, everything will make sense and your reward will come in a short time, in a surprising way.

This principle will bring you unimaginable benefits:

- It helps you organize and distribute your finances.
- It teaches you to consistently do what needs to be done.
- Someone will be blessed.

- There will be savings and reserve generation in your home.

- It will open the way for desired and planned investments.

- Allows you to use what is left over without guilt.

How to implement an efficient financial system

Now I know that you want to use this tool clearly, systematically and consistently. The result of this exercise - which involves your attention and work - will be the difference between getting desperate when the balance is zero and having to chase the money or looking in "your jar" for what is needed for payment or investment now.

This process doesn't require intellect or complex formulas to reach a common denominator and, much better: it works as an anxiety inhibitor. Every result will come from resting in the knowledge that your practice and obedience are subject to God's blessing, especially by virtue of your determination to pursue the blessing for your life. We can call this growth in wisdom.

The simplicity of the concept

The concept is simple, but it brings answers to the longings of the soul of people who may still be undecided about obedience and faith. And it's not about cheap spirituality just because we use the name of God in conjunction with finance. I may be redundant and insistent, but whenever something comes into your account or adds positively to your savings, be sure: do the exercise and separate everything into the five pots.

Over time, you'll be able to develop your own way of doing things. The manifold wisdom of the Holy Spirit will not prevent you from discovering other excellent tools drawn from the Word of God. The Holy Spirit is jealous of us because He knows that when we lose ourselves, His presence can be erased within us.

By adopting this practice, you don't just organize your finances and honor God with what He has given you; in fact, it works the other way around: first you honor and give God what is His and then your finances will be organized. Commit yourself to applying the principles of the Five Jars, transforming your financial life and experiencing prosperity that comes from God, by virtue of your obedience and commitment.

Preparing for financial success

How many times have you passed through a neighborhood in your city and seen beautiful houses for sale, but had to move on due to lack of resources? How many times have you passed up the option of realizing your dream home? What about that course you wanted to take but didn't have enough money to pay for? You thought: "Maybe next year I can do it!" What about your car, which is long past its sell-by date, but lack of savings prevents you from doing anything about it?

These are just a few examples of the many that illustrate the need to prepare so that your "emergencies" can be met calmly, without despair, without loans and, much better, without accumulating interest on interest. By preparing properly, you can face financial challenges with confidence and security.

The need for consistency

To do this, it is essential to correct one need - if it hasn't already been done - and that is consistency and seriousness in your decision to stick to what you have set as a priority. I say this because the temptation to use what you've multiplied on options that weren't planned will often appear with a twinkle in your eye and delight in your soul.

Although you will receive answers to the yearnings of the soul, the foundation of this principle is much more spiritual than you might think. And remember: the heart of man is deceitful. That's why your decision to follow the Five Jars tool must be so strong that it will resist the pressure of the waves of your will and the immediate desires of your heart.

Familiarity with the tool

A positive aspect of this tool is that you get used to it over time. Because it's something you do consistently, it becomes part of your culture. This new way of living will help you see your treasure growing gradually - whether in cents, tens, hundreds, thousands or millions. However, this only manifests itself with seriousness in application and the joy of doing what is right. The harder you work, and the more God allows you to earn, the more you will have the opportunity to accomplish what you set out to do. This is very important, because you don't want to see your castle collapse. This is the principle of this book: to present concepts that lead the reader to a healthy and multiplying lifestyle, if your heart and fear are in the Father's arms.

Responsibility for what we receive

Everything we have or receive doesn't fall into our hands by chance. If we have something or if we build something, we have an obligation to see it as a unique and exclusive opportunity - a gift that must be valued. It could be a hundred-dollar bill or the management of the most profitable company in town. The important thing is to understand and evaluate your mental, physical and spiritual health to touch and manage the "gift" that has come from God. That's why, in this principle, He must be the first in the whole process, both on the way out and on the way back.

The round-trip process

On the way out, whether you want to start your own business, if you're out of work or if you have an idea worth million, the tool is valid for everyone, because it starts with what you earn today or from today onwards.

On your return, when the results start to appear, it will be crucial to evaluate how your heart is, what you will do, how you will use it and how you will recognize all that you have received. This reflection is fundamental to ensure that you manage well the blessings that God has placed in your life and continue to grow in wisdom and prosperity.

Creating your protocols

So, here we go. When you get on an airplane, strict protocols are observed from start to finish so that it takes off and arrives at its destination. Do the same here and create your protocols; observe them and follow them to succeed in your endeavor.
I want to use the example of $1,000.00 (the currency you choose) to explain the modus operandi of this tool and how we can separate the values to achieve the desired multiplication. Imagine you have five jars in your hands. To make it clearer, you can make a table on your computer or cell phone, but the protocol is to separate them as I demonstrate below. Understanding this first step is fundamental.

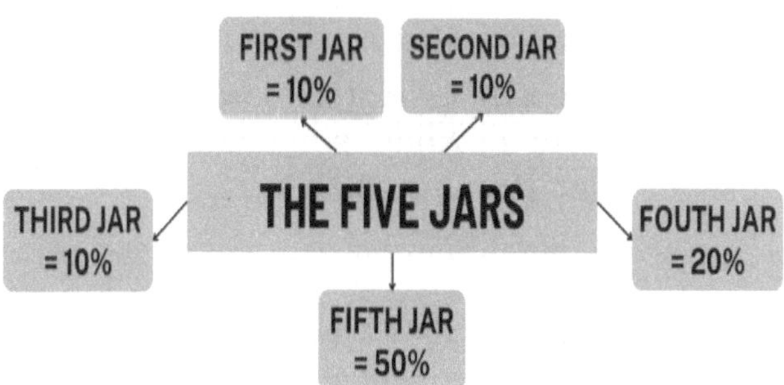

First Jar 10% (non-negotiable)

Pay attention to the words: "non-negotiable." What is not yours must be returned as soon as possible. If you keep what doesn't belong to you, knowing who it belongs to, that's what the Bible calls stealing. Separate and return to God what is His: the 10% (ten percent), which is your tithe. That's the first part, and God must be First in everything!
Get out of the concept and into a lifestyle that is consistent with your faith and your knowledge. If you have $1,000.00, set aside $100.00. Don't wait until Sunday or the next church meeting. Do it on the internet or PIX, whichever you prefer, but first and foremost, set aside what is the Lord's in this first jar. This is your best chance to learn how to manage what doesn't belong to you. I sacrifice the first so that the rest can be blessed.

> *"Consecrate to me every firstborn; every one that opens its mother's womb among the children of Israel, both man and beast, is mine."* [Exodus 13.2]

> *"Bring ye all the tithes into the treasury, that there may be meat in mine house: and prove me herewith, saith the Lord of hosts, if I will not open you the windows of heaven and pour you out a blessing without measure."* [Malachi 3.10]

"On the first day of the week, let each one of you set aside at home according to his prosperity, and gather, so that collections may not be made when I come." [1 Corinthians 16.2]

Second Jar 10% (negotiable)

In this jar, you set aside and bless someone or your church with another 10% (ten percent). The key here is generosity towards people, churches and projects. This 10% can be divided between the fronts you decide to support. How many times have you heard about something that needed to be done, corrected or fixed in the church? Or perhaps a missionary who is on a mission and has no way of earning a living the way you do? Or someone you know, or don't know, who needs financial support, however temporary? That's what offerings are for: to bless without expecting anything in return.
Here, you set aside another $100, pray and depend on the Holy Spirit to give you discernment about investing in people or projects. There will always be someone close to you who can be blessed.

Third Jar 10% (non-negotiable)

In this jar, you keep 10% (ten percent) of everything you receive. The examples I mentioned earlier - the beautiful house, the course you want or the car that needs changing - come into play here. By developing this habit repeatedly, without excuses or delays, you'll find it easier to cope with moments of crisis, such as an accident, the purchase of goods or other needs you consider important. This jar serves as an important step towards building your solid financial stability without unpleasant surprises. Set aside this $100.00 as savings for better days.

Fourth Jar **20%** (negotiable)

In this jar, you set aside 20% of everything you earn. Here, you make a real investment as an entrepreneur, where "two slices of this pizza" are exclusively set aside for what is your bigger vision. The focus is on multiplying and increasing your income. Give this dream a name and start giving thanks for this gift and the strategies that will be developed. Pray, make plans, draw, seek advice, research and set aside time to get to know and delve into the project you have chosen.

But be careful: if you intend to invest with other people, watch and pray. Check that these people are trustworthy and that they already have a good handle on what is placed in their hands. If they can't manage their own lives properly, how are they going to be any good in the business you propose and with your money? If you are married, this is the ideal time to share and decide with your spouse. At home, we always exchange ideas about investing in new businesses and, as well as praying, we need to be in full agreement before going ahead with the people we are thinking of working with. We've had problems because we didn't correctly discern between what was the will of God's Spirit or the anxiety of the soul.

This jar is negotiable because, if it is impossible to set aside 20% initially, adjust to a percentage that is increasing, scaling it up until you reach the desired percentage.

Don't give yourself room to settle and pursue your target as if it were your last step in the marathon of your dreams.

"Then he said, 'A certain nobleman set out for a distant land to take possession of a kingdom and return. He called ten of his servants, entrusted them with ten mines and said to them, 'Trade until I return. But his fellow citizens hated him and sent an embassy after him, saying: We don't want this one to reign over us. When he returned, having taken possession of the kingdom, he sent for the servants to whom he had given the money, to find out what business each of them had been able to do. The first came and said, "Sir, your mine has yielded ten. And the lord said to him, "Well done, good servant; because you have been faithful in a little, you will have authority over ten cities. The second came and said, "Sir, your mine has yielded five. To him he said, "You will have authority over five cities. Then another came, saying, "Sir,

here is your mina, which I kept wrapped in a handkerchief. For I was afraid of you, for you are a strict man; you take away what you have not put in, and you reap what you have not sown. He answered: You wicked servant, by your own mouth I will condemn you. You knew that I am a strict man, that I take away what I have not put in and reap what I have not sown; why didn't you put my money in the bank? Then, at my coming, I would receive it with interest. And he said to those who stood by, "Take the mina from him and give it to the one who has the ten. They said, "Sir, he already has ten. For I tell you, to everyone who has will be given; but from him who does not have, what he has will be taken away. But as for these my enemies, who did not want me to reign over them, bring them here and execute them in my presence." [Luke 19.12-27]

Fifth Jar 50% (negociável)

Now let's talk about the fifth jar. Note that even if you separate each of the four previous jars, you'll still have 50% of that amount left over. In the example we've given, you still have $500.00 (five hundred). This part of your finances goes towards paying your bills, going out with your family, guilt-free ice cream, extra shopping and enjoying entertainment, among other things.

The freedom of using the fifth jar

Don't be surprised! At first glance, it may seem a little daunting, especially if your bills are very tight. But remember: this jar is negotiable. So, work with the previous jar, using as little of the investment jar as possible until you can increase the percentage. For example, you can work to increase the investment jar from 20% to 25%, double your tithe, bless someone else in the second jar or save what's left over for times of greater need. Anything goes, if you are talking to and listening to the voice of the Holy Spirit.

Planning and flexibility

In the very near future, you may choose to have a fifth jar with 40% - or even less - and you can

increase the amounts in other jars. This flexibility is fundamental so that you can adapt your finances to your needs and goals over time. The important thing is that you feel comfortable and secure in how you are managing your resources.

By understanding and applying the Five Jars dynamic, you not only organize your finances, but also create a space to enjoy life without guilt. Remember that every part of your money has a purpose and, by using it wisely, you will invest in a prosperous and balanced future. May this practice become a natural part of your life, allowing you to live joyfully and generously, always honoring God in every financial decision you make.

Now, imagine yourself setting aside money every month using your financial income. Then add up what you could have in the next 12 months if you faithfully follow this tool. I'm sure you'll be surprised and very happy with the results.

Example of the 5 Jars

The 5 Jars Example with US$1,000.00/month			TOTAL 1 YEAR = 12 MONTHS
FIRST JAR	10%	US$ 100.00	US$ 1,200.00
SECOND JAR	10%	US$ 100.00	US$ 1,200.00
THIRD JAR	10%	US$ 100.00	US$ 1,200.00
FOUTH JAR	20%	US$ 200.00	US$ 2,400.00
	TOTAL JARS 1-4 = 50%	TOTAL JARS 1-4 = US$ 500.00	TOTAL JARS 1-4 = US$ 6,000
FIFTH JAR	50%	US$ 500.00	US$ 6,000.00
TOTAL:	100%	US$ 1,000.00	US$ 12,000.00
TOTAL:	100%	US$ 1,000.00	US$ 12,000.00

More strategies for managing your finances

For best results, try separating your money into separate accounts or create a table that allows you to visualize each action. You can open a file on your computer, make notes on your cell phone or use any other means you find convenient. Look at the example in the table above and fill it in with your own figures. This tool will not only make management easier but will also open space for your imagination.

The discernment of the Holy Spirit can take you much higher. Dedicate yourself to each of these steps with intensity and confidence until you realize that the gears are in motion and increasing their speed. From then on, your journey will become lighter, and you will soon begin to reap the rewards of this path - a real lifestyle!

Aim to work with focus and objectives. Your initial goal could be six months, followed by another six months. You'll soon find that a year of consistent, honest activity has given you results you've never experienced before. Celebrate every achievement!

"For which of you, intending to build a tower, does not first sit down to calculate the cost and see if he has the means to complete it?" [Luke 14.28].

Where is the treasure?

The secret lies in never using the money from one jar of provision, even if it is negotiable, to finance the activities of another jar without first discussing the strategy of this step - except in emergencies totally beyond your control. And if any negotiable jar needs changing, don't forget to establish criteria and follow them faithfully. Don't be like 96% of people who put off sorting out their investments to focus on their immediate needs. These people spend their lives on things that depreciate and become hostages to their own demands.

Meanwhile, only 4% of people work correctly, systematically and continuously, using and multiplying their earnings wisely. At the end of the day, these 4% of the world's society are the ones who don't take out loans, don't buy on crcdit and manage to see their money constantly multiplying, even when the job market is down.

The benefits of the Five Jars

What you learn from the Five Jars habit is impressive:

- You generate an attitude of respect for the things of God.

- Your financial habits are fully aligned with the Word.

- You establish legality in the lives of your children and an entire generation.

- You will always have enough in times of greatest instability.

- You can see your finances increase and multiply (everyone's dream);

- You will be able to fulfill everything the Bible sets out for God's children in a blessed way.

- You will have a debt-free life.

- You won't fall at the feet of the spirit of mammon.

- You will break the bonds of greed and lust.

- You will always have a financial margin.

- Generosity takes over!

Aligning faith and finances

By applying the principles shared here, you not only organize your finances, but also align your financial life with the teachings of God's Word. This generates a deep respect for the things of God and establishes a legality that can be passed on to future generations. This practice will guarantee you financial stability, even in the most challenging times. You will always have enough, and you will be able to watch your resources multiply, seeing your dreams come true. You will no longer be held hostage by debt or the spirit of mammon but will be able to walk free. Imagine this passing from father to son, from family to family, from generation to generation.

Generosity and blessings

By setting aside a percentage for offerings and projects, you will cultivate a generous heart. This generosity will not only bless others but will also come back to you in the form of unexpected blessings. You'll break the bonds of greed and usury, and you'll always have a financial margin to deal with unforeseen events.

Want more? Let God use you, brother!

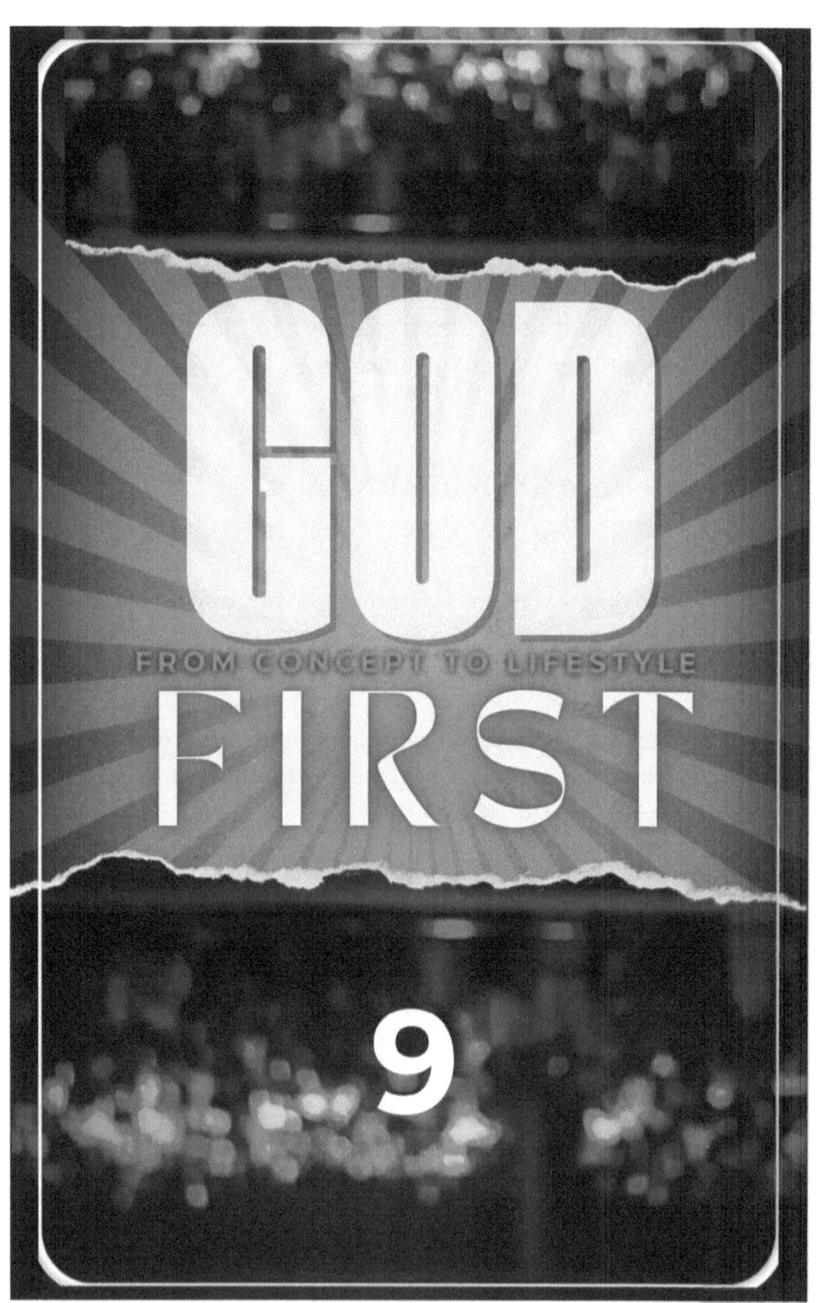

GOD
FROM CONCEPT TO LIFESTYLE
FIRST
9

9 - I'VE LEARNED THE CONCEPT, I WANT TO LIVE THE REALITY!

"...Do not be afraid. I am the First and the Last."
[Revelation 1.17]

This last chapter is not the end point; in fact, it's your starting point, your point of departure or maintenance! Join in this learning and start planning, always setting your priorities, investing in what you can and growing as a person. Prosperity, above all, is the result of a path where the first steps are generated through an intentional relationship with God. From this comes generosity and the spirit of a successful giver. Work to rescue what your parents couldn't hand down or teach you, and while you're at it, aim for your next generation to continue receiving the blessings you sought to share.

Setting clear objectives

To do this, set a clear goal. Your plan can be designed and refined from this reading; the ground is prepared, and your hands and heart are free to work. Seek to listen to the voice that speaks deepest in your spirit and become an example during so much filth spread around.

> *"Good people inherit for their grandchildren; the wealth of dishonest people ends up in the hands of the righteous."* [Proverbs 13.22]

Now it's up to you!

Evaluate your life with Christ, how much you trust Him and His Word, regardless of the circumstances that may arise - because they will always be present, in the most diverse forms. Evaluate your dreams and goals, as well as what you want to build and contribute as a legacy. Remember that circumstances produce people who are more attentive and sensitive, and it is these people who grow by winning their battles and looking firmly to the future that awaits them.

To give space to mammon, like people who feed their attention to this spirit, is to say that they do not love or worship God. Do your part as a giving heart and don't give way to the narcissistic spirit that plagues the world.

Walking with purpose

Always walk in the peace that fills your understanding, and not through emotions; rather, walk within the plan that you have prayed and designed, and manage it so that it is well executed. Don't walk like fools; take a serious look at the path of your financial inflows, from the smallest to the largest amount, from the inflows to the distribution of the money. Be faithful in the little, take good care of your obligations, and maintain this faithfulness when the little becomes much.

By following this path with purpose, you will build a solid foundation for your financial life. Remember that faithfulness in the small details is the key to achieving great things. Keep your focus on God, walk in obedience and allow Him to guide every step of your journey towards true prosperity.

The legacy you will build

Every person has a legacy. You have a legacy to establish; you are not so different from others, and you don't live in separate worlds. You live with struggles, doubts and inconsistencies, and you have choices to make. You can give up on everything, leave things as they are and live in complacency, or move forward, always fighting for your success.

I hope I have challenged you to grow and have the courage to act as an authentic Christian, who promotes the communication of the Gospel and declares who you are and who you believe in. Have the courage to be the Church that the world is waiting to see, without fear of continually delving deeper into Bible reading. Always maintain the tradition of gathering with your brothers and sisters and seek joy in the fundamentals you learned from your parents and teachers before you. This becomes a demonstration of courage and witness until you can say: "I am a Christian, come and follow me!" This was the way of life that Jesus presented.

My prayer for you

Lord God, thank you because you teach us so many principles and eternal truths that are not limited to today, to now, to here. Your truths teach us to be bigger and better. Lord, thank you because your Word is living and powerful, effective and capable of separating our thoughts, intentions and feelings. Help us, Father, so that the exercise of Your Word is more and more evident through our lives and that we are confronted, exercising with responsibility what we have in hand to do. May Your Word never return empty and forever fulfill Your purpose in what pleases You. It fulfills exactly the purpose that the Lord has planned for each one who reads this book and seeks, from the heart, to apply it. Amen.

The identity of a servant heart

You've already understood, but I need to say it again: Being rich is not the same as being prosperous. Being prosperous is a lifestyle that generates a personal identity that is always positive and aligned with God's precepts. The identity of a servant's heart that wants to please God. With this lifestyle, you'll be able to say: "I'm better today than I was then." May we all embrace this journey of growth and transformation, living fully the life God has for us!

"That's my promise, Lord!

I will spend my life to crown You!"

God bless you!

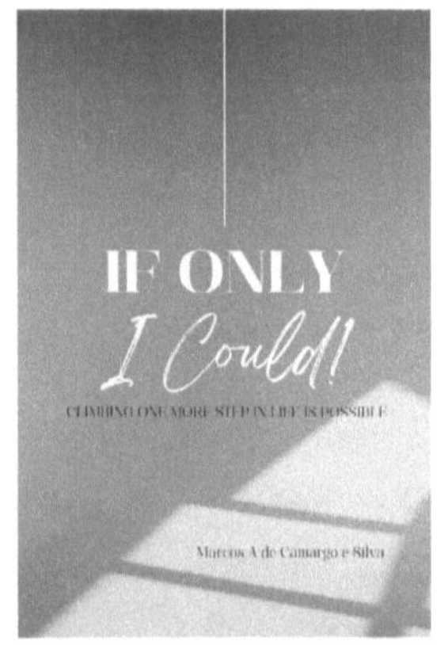
IF ONLY
I Could!
CLIMBING ONE MORE STEP IN LIFE IS POSSIBLE
Marcos A de Camargo e Silva

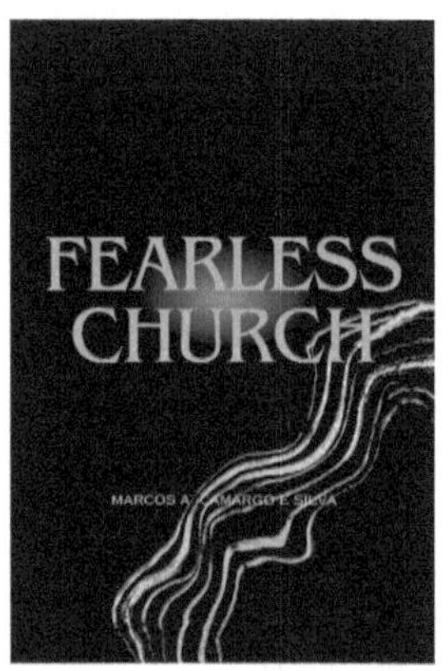
FEARLESS
CHURCH
MARCOS A CAMARGO E SILVA

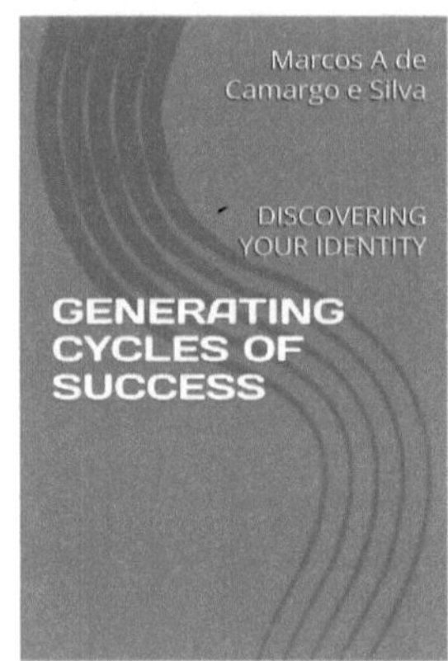
Marcos A de
Camargo e Silva

DISCOVERING
YOUR IDENTITY

GENERATING
CYCLES OF
SUCCESS

About the author:

Marcos A de Camargo e Silva is a member of APEL, Academia Paulista Evangélica de Letras. Senior Pastor of Igreja Deus Primeiro, in Barueri, SP, Brazil - Accredited by the International Coach Federation (PCC/ICF); Certified in Advanced Leadership by the Haggai Institute. He is currently president of DP Tranforma, an NGO focused on rescuing young people through sport (Jiu-Jitsu), through which he was a speaker at the 49th OAS Assembly (2019) in Colombia. He has a degree in Telecommunications from Oral Roberts University, Tulsa, Oklahoma; he was a visiting professor at Florida Christian University in Orlando, Florida. Founding partner of Willëm Books and Managing Partner of Coaching4Today's Leaders - Brazil Chapter (2002-2021).

...

Author of the books (distributed by Amazon.com):

- *When I Find Strength* (only in Portuguese)
- *Fearless Church*
- *Impossible is just a big word*
- *Haunted Heart*
- *If Only I Could*
- *God First - From Concept to Lifestyle*

Research material and references:

- (¹) (Van Inwagen, P. (1983). *An Essay on Free Will*. New York, NY: Oxford University Press.)
- (²) [Jeremiah.1.4]
- (³) [Psalms 139.1]
- (⁴) [James 4.13-14]
- (⁵) [James 4.10]
- (⁶) "When God Is First", Mike Hayes
- (⁷) a documentary by photographer Sebastião Salgado called *The Salt of the Earth*.
- (⁸) [2 Kings 5.15]
- (⁹) [2 Kings 5.20]
- (¹⁰) [Revelation 2.11; 3.5; 3:20; 21.6]
- (¹¹) God is at Work, Ken Eldred, pp.296, Regal.
- (¹²) Quando Deus é Primeiro, pg. 23, author: Mike Hayes, 2007, Editora Willem Books – Brasil.
- (¹³) Epicurus, Athenian philosopher of the 4th century BC.
- (¹⁴) Lei das Primícias, Luciano Subirá:
https://www.orvalho.com/ministerio/estudos-biblicos/a-lei-das-primicias-2/
- (¹⁵) *Cinco Segredos da Riqueza. Editora UDF, Craig Hill.* Brasil;
https://pt.slideshare.net/EmersonSouzaMBA/resumo-livro-cinco-segredos-da-riqueza
- Bíblia de Estudo NVT, Editora Mundo Cristão
- FREE WILL: https://carm.org/about-doctrine/if-god-is-all-knowing-and-he-knows-our-future-then-how-is-that-free-will/
https://closertotruth.com/video/if-god-knows-the-future-what-is-free-will/
- GIVE AND RECEIVE:
https://www.amberallen.com/uncategorized/the-law-of-giving-and-receiving/
https://www.linkedin.com/pulse/law-giving-receiving-bryan-daly-financial-head-coach
https://www.bethesdagardensthornton.com/blog/what-does-the-bible-say-about-giving-and-receiving
- Symbolism:
https://media.ascensionpress.com/2019/02/15/seven-examples-of-symbolism-in-the-bible/

www.ingramcontent.com/pod-product-compliance
Lightning Source LLC
Chambersburg PA
CBHW051253250726
48656CB00004B/1268